sleep

drink

breathe

sleep
drink
breathe

Simple Daily Habits for
Profound Long-Term Health

Michael Breus, PhD
THE SLEEP DOCTOR

LITTLE, BROWN SPARK

New York   Boston   London

Little, Brown Spark
Hachette Book Group
1290 Avenue of the Americas, New York, NY 10104
littlebrownspark.com

First Edition: December 2024

Little, Brown Spark is an imprint of Little, Brown and Company, a division of Hachette Book Group, Inc. The Little, Brown Spark name and logo are trademarks of Hachette Book Group, Inc.

The publisher is not responsible for websites (or their content) that are not owned by the publisher.

The Hachette Speakers Bureau provides a wide range of authors for speaking events. To find out more, go to hachettespeakersbureau.com or email hachettespeakers@hbgusa.com.

Little, Brown and Company books may be purchased in bulk for business, educational, or promotional use. For information, please contact your local bookseller or the Hachette Book Group Special Markets Department at special.markets@hbgusa.com.

Illustrations by Maggie Rosenberg

Print book interior design by Bart Dawson

ISBN 9780316576413
LCCN 2024942640

Printing 1, 2024

LSC-C

Printed in the United States of America

This book is dedicated to many people and one BIG idea: the Dominos of Wellness.

First, to my incredible family: Lauren, Cooper, and Carson, as well as our animals, who give so much joy — Mousse, aka Muffin, and Hugo, aka Sugar Bear. Book 6, and I'm still going strong. Couldn't do it without all of you.

Second, a special dedication to Dave Lakhani, may he rest in peace. Dave was one of my closest friends, as well as my mentor and business partner, who passed away unexpectedly in November 2022. I still miss you and talk to you in my head daily. Thank you for creating a safe place so I could have the confidence to take the biggest risks of my life, and for catching me when I failed. Not only did you help me build a business that helps millions of people every day, but you are still teaching me how to be a better human.

Finally, to all my patients who have all told me, "Wellness is too f*cking complicated!" I agree! This book is for you. Let's get back to the basics.

contents

INTRODUCTION: Wellness Is Too F*cking Complicated!   1

DOMINO ONE: SLEEP

CHAPTER 1: Sleep 411   17

CHAPTER 2: Sleep Assessment Tools   35

CHAPTER 3: Troubleshooting Sleep   49

CHAPTER 4: Sleep for the Win   75

DOMINO TWO: DRINK

CHAPTER 5: Drink 411   97

CHAPTER 6: Drink Assessment Tools   109

CHAPTER 7: Troubleshooting Drink   123

CHAPTER 8: Drink for the Win   139

DOMINO THREE: BREATHE

CHAPTER 9: Breathe 411   165

CHAPTER 10: Breathe Assessment Tools   177

CHAPTER 11: Troubleshooting Breathe   187

CONTENTS

CHAPTER 12: Breathe for the Win   205

CHAPTER 13: The Sleep-Drink-Breathe Nexus   235

THE SLEEP-DRINK-BREATHE PLAN   241

ACKNOWLEDGMENTS   271
NOTES   273
INDEX   297

introduction

Wellness Is Too F*cking Complicated!

Does this sound familiar: You listened to your favorite wellness or health podcast and bought a month's worth of "green juice" they recommended, which tasted so bad that you never drank more than a sip. Or you installed a cold plunge in your yard and sat in it once. Or you invested in supplements (expensive ones) that promised to "optimize" every system in your body, but they ended up gathering dust on the shelf. Your Peloton turned into a clothes rack. Your plan to eat only non-GMO, whole food meal kits wound up eating through your savings, with zero benefits to show for it.

As the Sleep Doctor, I see and speak to a multitude of health enthusiasts in every major field, and I have the same conversation in some form or fashion ten times a day. Lately, the conventional wisdom says you must read every article and try every new technique, supplement, or gizmo in order to be well, but you end up just feeling lost because the trendy supplements and methods change so frequently that you don't even know if what you are doing is still recommended.

Not to mention the expense! A lot of wellness products and programs put health at a premium, behind a paywall. Wellness influencers and podcasters have turned health into a luxury industry.

Despite what they might have you believe, good health *is* accessible to everyone—free! You don't need to buy all the things, no matter what the super fit and "well" people say on social media. It's also not your fault for being drawn into the wellness vortex. It's pervasive in our culture. And who can resist the idea of some new biohack that is going to prevent or cure any ill?

What if I told you that most of the health conscious among us are approaching wellness the *wrong* way? By trying the latest, greatest techniques and grasping for an ambiguous state of wellness, people forget about the most basic aspects of good health. By thinking they need to Do It All and start "new year, new me" intense, whole-life changes in January, they fall short because it's too much change, too fast. They get overwhelmed. Frustration and guilt set in, and they give up...until the next hot trend comes along.

You don't need to keep up with trends or suffer from wellness FOMO. If you just get down the basics, the DNA of health, you can reset the body and create an internal environment that promotes good health at zero or low cost. The truth is, there are a few simple bodily functions or biobehaviors that you *must* do every day, multiple times a day. If you can get those correct, general wellness will result.

Imagine if I told you the secret to real, long-lasting wellness came down to the number three (a number I happen to have an affinity for—it just feels manageable). The big three essential, whole-body impactful and adjustable biobehaviors are as follows: sleeping, drinking (hydrating), and breathing. If *everyone* just focused on these three things, before exploring all the gizmos, gadgets, lotions, and potions in the wellness space, they would find themselves at the starting line for overall health, and they would not be intimidated (as I was, and so many are) by the sheer volume of information and expensive products that promise revolutionary results.

So let me ask you a very simple question:

What if you are sleeping, drinking, and breathing wrong?

Is that even a thing?

You bet!

Doctors rarely talk about these behaviors at your annual wellness visit. Your primary care physician *might* ask, "How are you sleeping?" or "Are you drinking enough water?" But I'd fall off the exam table if they asked, "How deep are your breaths?" Unless you are at high risk for respiratory illness, a smoker, or already diagnosed with chronic obstructive pulmonary disease (COPD), the subject would likely *never* come up.

Sleeping, drinking, and breathing—three life-sustaining biobehaviors—are given little attention by primary care doctors because they assume the patient must be doing them well enough or they wouldn't be able to walk into the office.

That's what I think most people are doing when it comes to sleeping, drinking (hydrating), and breathing.

Let's be honest, doctors take patients' fundamental proficiency in these three basics for granted. And you probably do the same thing. You might even be thinking right now, *Why do I need to worry about this? I've been sleeping, drinking, and breathing my whole life, and I've gotten this far. Besides, my body handles all that for me automatically.*

Doing something *adequately,* or at the bare minimum, is not the same as doing it well and getting more out of your effort. When it comes to the fundamentals for your health, wellness, and longevity, if you are going to be sleeping, hydrating, and breathing anyway, why not get the most out of it by learning a few simple habits that lead to profound improvements? Think about it like this: You already know how to walk; if you take 10,000 steps per day, then walking will do you much more good!

To the second point—i.e., why you should worry about your proficiency in biobehaviors that are automatically regulated—it is true that your body has systems in place to put you to sleep, make you thirsty so you drink, and keep your lungs inhaling and exhaling. Here's a quick rundown on those systems:

Sleeping. The body's watchdog for sleep and most biological functions is the circadian master clock, a bundle of nerves called the suprachiasmatic nucleus (SCN), located in the hypothalamus, an almond-sized gland buried deep in your brain. When it gets dark outside, the SCN signals the pineal gland to start the slow release of the hormone melatonin, which sets off a chain reaction that shuts off production of the stress hormone cortisol and lowers blood pressure, body temperature, and heart rate so you can relax into rest and sleep. The same process in reverse—melatonin stops, cortisol secretions surge, and blood pressure, body temperature, and heart rate go up—is what wakes you up in the morning.

Drinking. Your thirst command center is also located in the hypothalamus. It keeps tabs on the all-important water-to-salt ratio in your blood. When sodium concentration gets too high, the hypothalamus sends out signals to nerves in the mouth and throat that create the sensation of thirst. Suddenly, you crave water. If you don't drink, your body reminds you to do it via a parched throat, dry mouth and lips, dry eyes, irritability, perhaps even a headache. If you ignore those signals, your brain will send emergency alerts. Symptoms will intensify until you take a long gulp or three . . . and while you are enjoying a hydrating beverage, your brain will give you a hit of dopamine as a little thank-you gift.

Breathing. The continuous inhaling and exhaling we do between 17,000 and 25,000 times per day is controlled and monitored by our autonomic nervous system (ANS), the same system that keeps our hearts beating, guts digesting, and livers metabolizing. Our bodies perform these life-sustaining functions for us without our having to remember to do them. When's the last time you made a mental note, "Must not forget to tell lungs to breathe deeply when I sprint"? Nope. It just happens, whether or not you think about it.

The respiratory center that oversees breathing is located in the brain's medulla oblongata. It vigilantly monitors the ratio of oxygen to carbon dioxide in your blood. If it detects too much CO_2, it signals to the intercostal muscles between the ribs and the diaphragm muscle in the abdomen to contract, which forces air out of the lungs. In need of O_2, the brain tells the rib muscles to spread and the diaphragm to flatten, causing the lungs to expand. This action creates a vacuum effect that draws air through the nose and mouth (we will talk about nose vs. mouth breathing later), down the windpipe, and into the tiny air sacs in the lungs.

Your body truly is a marvel. It's doing all this, and *so much more*, that you have little or no conscious awareness of. When all your organs and systems are working at peak efficiency, together in harmony, you are in a state called homeostasis, or whole-body balance. However, homeostasis is delicate. You could just go on with your life, taking your regulatory systems for granted, assuming your body will achieve homeostasis no matter what you do. But that would be a mistake.

The brain's fail-safes that monitor sleeping, hydrating, and breathing can be disrupted by stress, technology, light pollution, environmental and food toxins, anxiety, too much sitting, caffeine, alcohol, drugs — basically *modern life*. Within the context of modern existence, our most basic bodily functions get complicated and, often, compromised.

Even just a small glitch in any of your life-sustaining, fundamental biobehaviors can set off a cascade of bad reactions that throws your entire system out of whack, creating chaos that can result in disease-causing inflammation, weight gain, hormonal imbalance, emotional swings, and low energy.

Chaos, like balance, is not permanent. By tweaking things you're already doing—like sleeping, drinking water, and breathing—you can trigger a beneficial cascade of *good* reactions that gets you back into the internal harmony of homeostasis. You can rebalance hormones, decrease inflammation, increase energy and calm, improve quality of life, and decrease the risk of illness and death, practically overnight.

The body wants to be in balance. It wants to feel good. You just have to help it do what it wants to do. Humans have the power to live well, to go beyond just surviving. By shoring up the fundamentals, we can thrive. We *can* be the TSwizzle of sleep, the Gordon Ramsay of hydration, the Steph Curry of breathing, one night, one glass of water, one breath at a time.

THE DOMINOS OF WELLNESS

Every action affects and causes other actions. One faulty behavior leads to others, and the consequences aren't necessarily just doubled; they're often multiplied.

But the good news is the opposite is also true: One healthy behavior leads to others, and the exponential rewards can change the course of your life.

I have seen this phenomenon play out countless times in my twenty-four years as an actively practicing sleep doctor. When patients establish a healthy sleep routine, they are more energized throughout the day, and they make better choices about almost everything. Smarter snack options. More gym visits. Positive change isn't limited to health. When brain fog clears, people start crushing it at work. If they're well rested and less irritable, their relationships improve. By fixing one broken biobehavioral process, so many other surprising aspects of one's mental, emotional, and physical health improve, as if on their own. One patient said to me, "Who knew that sleeping better would get me a raise and stop my divorce proceedings?"

Reflecting on this, I started to think of good sleep as the first domino in a long line of others. Wellness starts with utterly basic behaviors. So good sleep is the first domino in a line of them. Once you get that one "down," other benefits and behaviors will go down...and you know what happens next. Your body is on a path to reaching your wellness goals, whatever that means for you. Your goals could be a healthy diet, regular exercise, reduced inflammation, lowered stress, and a happier mindset, to name a few. By knocking down the domino of sleep, the rest can topple, too, with minimal effort. At the end of the line of toppled dominos, you'd find what we all want: a balanced internal environment that is the basis of good health, wellness, and happiness. I used to tell my patients, "If you get sleep down, it sets off a beneficial chain reaction. It causes so many other behaviors that lead to good health falling into place without your really having to do anything else."

I began referring to sleep as the "Domino of Wellness" after reading a book by my dear friend Joe Polish, called *Life Gives to the Giver.* In it, he describes the concept of fundamental dominos for many areas of life. I asked myself, "What would the fundamental dominos of wellness be, because this has just gotten too f*cking complicated?!"

Along with seeing positive results among my patient population, I looked into the science as well. Since I do like to nerd out, I dug into the literature to confirm my theory and found a mountain of evidence that backs it up. If humans optimize the essential biobehavior of sleep, their overall health and wellness—their entire life—benefits.

According to the 2023 National Sleep Foundation poll, using its Best Slept Self ratings system of good sleep health, 75 percent of the population received C, D, or F grades. Roughly the same percentage reported low sleep satisfaction.[1] As a result, millions are suffering from lowered immunity, exhaustion, chronic inflammation, cognitive issues, mood disorders, and so much more.

Sleep is Domino One. Sleep is my primary area of expertise, the first fundamental biobehavior to fix so you can reap the rewards.

Hydration is Domino Two. I don't have a degree in hydration, but as a lifelong runner and fitness guy, I have made a careful study of it. I'm a heavy sweater. If I run one mile, my entire shirt is drenched. So I have been researching hydration for years and incorporating that study into my clinical work. What I've learned is that 75 percent of Americans are chronically dehydrated.[2] A dehydrated body, and the sluggish circulatory system that goes with it, is unable to efficiently deliver nutrients to organs and cells. Its hormonal pathways are jammed. Recent research links dehydration with chronic inflammation, which we have heard about nonstop for the last several years as the cause of so many illnesses, including diabetes, arthritis, heart conditions, and stroke. On the other hand, a well-hydrated body can brim with energy, immunity, and well-fed cells.

Breathing is Domino Three. For the first six and a half years after my doctorate, I worked in a medical clinic, Southeastern Lung Care in Decatur, Georgia, with a staff of six pulmonologists. My focus was on sleep apnea, a breathing disorder. In that environment, working side by side with my colleagues, I learned quite a bit about breathing, and have augmented that knowledge outside clinical and academic pursuits by training with experts such as Wim Hof and attending breathwork retreats. What I've learned is that most of us don't know how to breathe. That might sound ridiculous. After all, we all do it between six and twenty-five times per minute. Larger adults have the lung capacity to take in six liters of air with every breath, but most of us are reaching only 70 percent of that, even when we're young. As people age, lung function rapidly declines by as much as 40 percent.[3] To slow the downward trend, people need to strengthen respiratory muscles. When's the last time you gave a second's thought to toning your diaphragm? What's more, by exercising the lungs and accompanying muscles, you tone the vagus nerve — one of the longest nerves in the body, which stretches from brain stem to pelvis and influences nearly every organ in between. Critically, the vagus nerve activates the parasympathetic nervous system (aka the rest-and-digest system), turning off the stress response so you can switch into relaxation mode for healing and rejuvenation. That sounds like the ticket to wellness, for sure.

As I said, all good health begins with homeostasis. But...

You can't reach whole-body balance without sleeping, drinking, and breathing optimally.

Balance is attainable by tinkering with sleeping, drinking, and breathing habits. You don't have to buy a $5,000 mattress or a $45 Stanley water bottle. The changes I'm talking about are little things that anyone can do, *free*. As soon as you start wobbling the three Dominos of Wellness, you'll feel better as you go through your day, with more energy and a positive outlook. Meanwhile, inside your body, inflammation will recede. Hormones will balance. And cells will rejoice. Sleep, drink, and breathe your way to reaching your wellness goals. Then you can decide about green drinks, saunas, cold plunges, and whatever other new idea pops on the market.

To enjoy the Domino of Wellness effect, you need to learn about the three systems, unlearn some bad habits, and establish some new ones. I've organized this book to optimize how you take in the information so you can use it to your advantage. For each domino, you will get:

- **The 411**, or the simple facts. It's not enough to just tell you what to do. If you understand the "why," you're more likely to follow through on the "how." I'm going to explain how sleep, hydration, and breathing work, and what they do internally, so that you have the knowledge to get the dominos *down*. Don't worry. I won't go off too deep or use confounding language. I'm here to simplify, not overwhelm.
- **Assessment Tools**. All improvement paths start with a baseline measurement of the right metrics. How are you doing now as a sleeper, drinker, and breather? I'll walk you through at-home low- or no-cost tests to get answers. Once you have a baseline, you can steadily improve upon it as you knock down each domino.
- **Troubleshooting**. I'll show you the consequences of suboptimal sleep, hydration, and breathing, and discuss what you might need to change. It's about motivation and information, not shame. Unlearn before you relearn. I will also point out solutions to some of the top issues people have during this period of relearning.
- **Optimization**. I'll give you only the best methods and practices, based on real science — as well as recommendations for technology — so you can establish new habits and knock down dominos quickly.

HOW TO USE THIS BOOK

If you are a health-conscious person, you might think you know everything about some of these topics. But I'm providing a ton of information here, and it's highly likely you will learn something new, even in an area that's familiar to you. That said, if you think that you've got the sleep domino down already, you can skim the sleep chapters, maybe take one assessment, and then just move on to the hydration section. Or jump straight to breathing assessment tools. Or go right to hydration troubleshooting. It's kind of a choose-your-own-adventure experience, based on what you need. You might want to read it cover to cover. (If you do, you'll have all the information, and that will help reinforce the recommendations.) Or you might want to skip ahead to the Sleep-Drink-Breathe Plan at the end, familiarize yourself with it, and then go back to the educational chapters later. However you choose to use this book is just fine.

As a licensed healthcare professional, I can tell you that the biggest obstacle to patients' positive outcomes is compliance, or follow-through. From what I've seen, people struggle with following doctors' advice if it's too complicated. Well, there's no choice when it comes to compliance here. You *must* do these three biobehaviors every day. And if you must do them, you might as well do them right.

To make compliance as easy as possible, I've taken all the science and turned it into a simple plan for toppling the three Dominos of Wellness every day.

The Sleep-Drink-Breathe Plan, which you can find at the end of the book, is a three-week regimen that seamlessly incorporates the strategies for optimal sleep, hydration, and breathing into your life. I think of it as a summary, in which established science meets common sense.

The plan is perfectly simple, and easy to implement. At first, you'll incorporate just a few changes into your life at a time, and then you'll add a couple more. As you change your behavior, you'll notice improvement in energy and mood immediately, and that will keep you motivated to keep going. All the adaptations are easy and pleasant. In fact, you will come to look forward to each action item in this plan and maybe even feel strange if you don't do it.

Because the Sleep-Drink-Breathe Plan is so straightforward, you won't be intimidated by it and you will stick with it. After just a few days, you'll feel better physically, mentally, and emotionally. After a few weeks, you will have established new, healthier habits and retrained the brain to make them automatic. You can go back to not thinking about the Dominos of Wellness again, with the confidence that you're now doing them right. Or maybe you want to tell a loved one, family member, or friend about how easy this process really is—then maybe you will become the "realistic healthy friend" to those around you.

After a month or two, as you breeze through life, you'll realize, "Hey, I haven't had a cold in a long time." Curveballs that used to ruin your day you will take in stride. You will do the crossword puzzle in less time. You will stop craving junk food. You will have more energy and spend less time sitting around. The waist of your jeans may be looser.

> *Most of the wellness problems people dwell on seem to take care of themselves when they optimize the simple things first.*

I keep using the word *simple* for a reason. Good health doesn't have to be complicated. There's so much noise out there about how to be well. It's my job to keep up with this stuff, and even *I* feel over-whelmed by all the chatter about macros, microbiomes, calorie defi-cits, HIIT training... the list seems endless.

People need to stop worrying so much about combining inter-mittent fasting with counting protein grams and servings of green drinks.

Wellness begins with the basics. You can reach your wellness goals by tweaking three biobehaviors you're already doing, and then the rest will either happen automatically or be substantially easier to reach.

It's deeper than "You have to crawl before you can walk." By knocking down the sleep, drink, and breathe dominos with consis-tency, you will feel like you have brand-new legs.

The first domino to get down is sleep. No need to hit the snooze. Let's get right into it.

TO-DO'S

- **Reset your thinking about wellness.** It's not about gizmos and complicated plans. It's about focusing on fundamentals and getting the basics right.
- **Don't take sleeping, drinking (hydration), and breathing for granted.** Yes, your body has regulatory systems in place, but life causes all kinds of glitches.
- **Get those Dominos of Wellness down.** Sleep, hydration, and breathing are the three Dominos of Wellness you'll master in this book. For now, embrace the idea that simple actions can create profound changes in your health and wellness.

- **Make whole-body balance your top wellness goal**. When all your systems work in harmony, your health goals will be within reach. Sleeping, hydrating, and breathing well are the fastest, best ways to get back into whole-body balance.

DOMINO ONE

sleep

Simplify health and wellness by getting
the first fundamental biobehavior down.

CHAPTER 1

Sleep 411

> Perhaps it's time to wake up to the fact that if you
> spend one third of your entire life doing something,
> you need to know more about it. In this chapter,
> I'll answer some questions you might have about sleep,
> and some you've never thought to ask.

WHAT EXACTLY IS SLEEP?

WHY DO PEOPLE SLEEP?

HOW DO YOU FALL ASLEEP?

WHAT HAPPENS WHEN YOU'RE ASLEEP?

WHAT ARE DREAMS?

CAN NOT SLEEPING KILL YOU?

**WHAT HAPPENS TO YOU IF YOU'RE SEVERELY
SLEEP-DEPRIVED?**

A note from Dr. B: If you have skipped the book's introduction, please do me the favor of going back and reading it. It will really help you understand the entire program and how it can drastically improve your life through small, daily changes!

Thank you!

In the past ten years the number of cases of sleep disorders has risen significantly, with insomnia rates increasing in the double digits.[1] Once COVID-19 hit, basically all hell broke loose, in terms of sleep. Per the results of a 2022 survey about sleep habits during the pandemic, published in *Sleep Science*[2]:

- Seventy percent of study respondents reported sleep disturbances.
- Eight percent reported symptoms of anxiety, which disrupted sleep.
- Sleep duration decreased from about seven hours per night to around six.
- Sleep dissatisfaction increased 28 percent.
- Complaints about difficulty falling asleep increased by more than 30 percent.

These results are extreme. The population surveyed was largely healthcare workers who in many cases faced increased work-related stress during the COVID-19 years. But the general population experienced unusual stressors during the pandemic, too, which also affected sleep. And it isn't just sleep disorders that are stacking up. What I call Disordered Sleep—when sleep does not quite qualify you for a formal sleep disorder, but when you wake up, after six, seven, or eight hours, and still feel like crap—is on the rise as well.

Why is our sleep so disordered? What leads to the fundamental problem of not getting good quality sleep? In a word: education.

People are barely taught about sleep in school — including medical school. Most of us have never learned about the mechanics of sleep or answers to the most basic questions, like "What is sleep?" and "What happens when I'm asleep?" Without essential knowledge and appreciation, it's no wonder people think that they can be fully functional on five hours of sleep per night or that extreme fatigue can be powered through with Red Bull.

Sorry, but no. To get this domino down, you need the truth. And who better to give it to you, than me, the Sleep Doctor?

WHY DO PEOPLE SLEEP?

Scientists know a lot about the benefits of sleep for mental and physical health. There is even a book titled *Why We Sleep* (which never seems to answer the question), but I'd be lying if I said that the scientific community had complete clarity on why humans evolved to spend seven or eight hours per day unconscious. It doesn't seem practical when we have so much to do.

There are some theories that make sense. Taken as a whole, they add up to a comprehensive (but as yet incomplete) explanation of why we sleep.[3]

The Energy Conservation Theory. People think sleep is a shutting down, like turning off a computer. That's a misconception. Your body is energized even when you're asleep. The only time you don't have any energy is when you're dead. Sleep is more like energy transfer with a slight decrease in intensity — like putting your computer into power-saving mode. During most stages of sleep, the body uses less energy, but it's still "on." Metabolism decreases overnight, but only by 10 percent.[4] According to scientists at the

University of Colorado, Boulder, sleep is likely to be a "physiological adaptation to conserve energy."[5] The body saves up energy overnight so you have the get-up-and-go in the morning to hunt your metaphorical mammoth.

> **Sleep Science:** I encourage my patients to conceptualize sleep as an energy transfer. Falling asleep is transferring energy in a different direction – away from answering emails and toward rhythmic breathing, for example. When my patients focus on enacting this transfer themselves, they go down faster and have higher-quality rest.

The Restorative Theory. When in deep sleep, you appear inactive because you mostly just lie there. But you're really in an active state of unconsciousness. It sounds like an oxymoron, but it's not. The central point to understand is that you are *always* biologically busy, but your body and brain do different things at different times, depending on whether you're conscious or unconscious.

When conscious, your cells are busy with the tasks of the day: moving, metabolizing, digesting, thinking, releasing hormones. You are a human machine. And like all machines with many cogs and functions, some parts are bound to degrade with use. Cellular wear-and-tear is totally normal.

When unconscious, your body and brain go about the tasks of restoring and repairing cells that have broken down over the course of the day. Growth hormone secretions peak at night,[6] rushing in to repair muscles, tissues, and bones. In a 2021 Italian study of patients who'd suffered rotator cuff tears on their shoulders and then underwent corrective surgery, researchers found that sleep quality significantly affected the recovery process.[7]

Better sleep meant faster healing. During sustained sleep (not the fragmented kind when you wake up in the middle of the night and can't fall back to sleep), certain genes activate stem cells that prevent age-related deterioration.[8]

Sleep brings you the gift of regeneration on the cellular level. From an evolutionary standpoint, we need hours of unconsciousness every day to fix our fragile human bodies. Otherwise, our species would never have survived for so long.

The Brain Plasticity Theory. The human brain is a fast learner and ruthless editor. We have a near unlimited capacity to take in, store, and process new information. The brain blazes new neural pathways between synapses as fresh data comes in. But if data becomes extraneous, the brain prunes away neural pathways that you no longer need or use. Neuroplasticity—the brain's ability to mold itself as we learn and change—happens 24/7. But brain circuitry looks and functions differently depending on our conscious or unconscious state. During waking hours, it blazes and prunes. During sleep, it cleans up the mess left behind by all that blazing and pruning. We need both growth while awake and repair while asleep to process and store memories.[9] Sleep allows the brain to adapt. Paraphrasing Charles Darwin, strength and intelligence are all well and good. But the ability to adapt is the key to species survival and success.

HOW DO YOU FALL ASLEEP?

My insomnia patients ask me this question every day. On a purely biological level, there are two separate processes that help us create sleep: sleep drive and sleep rhythm.

Sleep drive. This mechanism promotes sleep and controls the intensity of it. A good comparison to sleep drive is hunger. If you go a long time without food, you get hungrier and hungrier throughout the day. When you finally dig in, that gnawing "I'm starving!" feeling fades away. The same holds true for sleep. The longer you go without it, the greater your desire for it. That eyelids-drooping "I'm exhausted" feeling is your sleep drive nagging you to go to bed. The feeling may come and go, but the longer you go without sleep, the worse it gets.

Biologically speaking, the drowsy feeling is caused by the buildup of the chemical adenosine in the brain. Adenosine is a byproduct of cellular metabolism. Just as you eat food, digest it, and produce waste, your cells do the same on a much smaller scale. To keep all your systems going throughout the day, cells gobble up glucose, metabolize it (convert it into energy), and, in that process, produce adenosine. Along with other metabolic byproducts, adenosine is dumped into the bloodstream. It travels to the brain and latches on to specific receptor sites. As those receptor sites fill up, you become more and more tired. When you sleep, adenosine is washed out of the brain. You wake up and start the sleep-drive-cycle of daytime adenosine buildup and nighttime clearing all over again.

Sleep rhythm. We all have a twenty-four-hour master clock in the brain that tells the body when it's time to do and feel pretty much everything. You have undoubtedly noticed that you get hungry at particular times throughout the day. Your circadian rhythm for feeding rings the meal bell due, in part, to the timely release of the hunger hormone ghrelin. You have an internal clock that tells you to feel tired after darkness falls because the pineal gland releases melatonin, which makes you yawn, and the adrenal gland stops secreting the stimulating hormone cortisol. Those changes mean it's getting close to bedtime. In the morning, as first light enters your eyes and pings your optic nerve, the master clock in the hypothalamus starts the wake-up process. Blood pressure and body temperature go up, melatonin ebbs, and cortisol flows.

Serotonin and gamma-aminobutyric acid (GABA)[10] are also involved, but cortisol serves as nature's primary alarm clock, nudging you awake. And the sleep rhythm cycle begins again.

When your sleep drive is elevated and your sleep rhythm is in sync, you will usually fall asleep within fifteen minutes and sleep well throughout the night. When either of these are off, that is when you can be diagnosed with a sleep disorder.

> *Sleep Science*: You went on a hike, worked in your garden, or did a vigorous workout. You are tired, so you decide to go to bed early (like 8:00 p.m.) and one of two things happens when you get in bed. Either you fall asleep and then wake up one to two hours later and are wide awake for the rest of the night, or you just lie there staring at the ceiling, feeling physically exhausted, but also wired and perhaps pissed off.

WHAT EXACTLY IS SLEEP?

In the simplest terms, **sleep is a vital, natural, biological process** that allows the brain and body to rest, recover, recharge, and heal.

It's a period of unconsciousness when you are unaware of what's happening around you. But unlike other states of unconsciousness, caused, for instance, by excessive alcohol use or being in a coma, sleep is relatively easy to come out of.

It's partly involuntary. The body has mechanisms in place to promote sleep—like the release of the melatonin when it gets dark and the corresponding drop in cortisol—but you can't make yourself fall asleep the way you can snap your fingers. And while you can make yourself stay awake to a point, you can also fall asleep without wanting or trying to.

It's both a universal and an individual experience. What I find fascinating about sleep is that we all have a unique experience with it. Everyone sleeps, but no two people pass their nocturnal journey in exactly the same way. And yet, the mechanics and architecture of the biological process are pretty much the same for each of us.

> **My Sleep Story**: In my many years of lecturing around the globe, I think the best definition I've heard came when I was speaking to a group of preschool kids: "Sleep is when your body goes into healing and adventure mode and when Mommy and Daddy get time to kiss."

WHAT HAPPENS WHILE YOU'RE ASLEEP?

During unconsciousness, your body and brain are repaired and restored to factory settings so you begin each day reset and ready. Sleep is like taking your car into the repair shop each night to buff away the scratches and dings and vacuum up the cellular trash and toxins, leaving it shiny and clean from the inside out in the morning.

Within that repair shop, there are four rooms, or "stages." Each has its own look, in terms of brain activity and body state. And each one is dedicated to different aspects of restoration.

Stage 1, the transition from waking to very light sleep, a brief dozing-off portion of the night. This stage can be like skipping a stone on a lake, skimming the surface tension of sleep before dropping into it. As your body relaxes, you might have the unpleasant feeling of suddenly falling and then jerking back awake. Those sensations are caused by muscle contractions known as hypnic jerks. (The sensation of falling makes me think we're literally "falling" asleep.) When any such jerking stops and you drift off, muscle activity slows. Stage 1 usually lasts about ten minutes, or 2 to 3 percent of your night. Most trackers will lump this into "light sleep" and then you move into . . .

Stage 2, the transitional period between light and deeper sleep. During this stage, eye movement stops and brain waves slow way down, except for occasional fast brain activity bursts called "sleep spindles," which are important for sensory processing and memory. Muscles continue to relax and the heart rate decreases. This makes up the bulk of the night (50 percent, in some cases even more) and is also lumped in with light sleep on all trackers. After up to twenty-five minutes of this, you plunge into . . .

Stage 3, deep, restful sleep. Everything drops: respiration rate, heart rate, blood pressure. Brain waves slow and spread out in a Delta pattern. Eye movement and muscle activity stop. You are "out." To wake someone during this stage, you'd need to shake them pretty hard. And when they woke up, they'd feel groggy and disoriented, like "Where am I?" for a few minutes.

The major benefit of Stage 3 is full-body restoration and healing. Your immune system goes into overdrive, attacking infection-causing bacteria and viruses and stepping up production of human growth hormone to regenerate and repair cells. This stage lasts for up to forty minutes. In the past, sleep scientists had another category, stage 4, of deep sleep, but as seen in sleep laboratories, peoples' brain waves jump back and forth between stages 3 and 4 so much that they were combined into one stage, often called N3.

Typically, after a visit to Stage 3, you backtrack to Stage 2, and from there, you zoom ahead into REM sleep.

REM is a state of deep sleep with increased brain activity. Breathing becomes rapid, irregular, and shallower. Heart rate and blood pressure tick back up to wakefulness levels. And yet, despite increased pulse and respiration, muscles are paralyzed during REM.

25

Eye movements become rapid, jerking around in all directions like pinballs. If you wake up during REM, you might remember your dreams, which are more vivid than in any other stage. The big benefit of REM is mental and emotional restoration and memory consolidation. If you've ever gone to bed pissed off about something and woken up the next day thinking, "It's not nearly as bad as I thought last night," you can thank REM for separating the upsetting memory from the intense feelings you experienced during the event that made you angry.[11] During this stage, the brain makes sense of the events of the day, contextualizes them based on past experiences, learns from them, and sorts and stores them in the correct filing cabinets in your mind.[12] So much gets done, yet this stage lasts for just sixty minutes, max.

> **Sleep Science**: The glymphatic system is the brain's dedicated trash removal service. Starting during Stage 3 and continuing in REM, cerebrospinal fluid floods into the brain, delivering nutrients (glucose, lipids, and amino acids) it needs to function, while simultaneously power-washing away neurotoxic waste products (like beta amyloid and tau) accumulated during the day. Once it's flushed out your brain, the dirty cerebrospinal fluid drains into your lymphatic system and is eventually transported out of the body via urine.

After a REM session is complete, you might wake up for several seconds and then drift back into Stage 1 to begin again.

The process of moving through all four stages (including normal backtracking) is called a "sleep cycle." Cycles are shorter early in the night, lasting from 70 to 100 minutes. As the night progresses, cycles get longer, lasting from 90 to 120 minutes, with a greater percentage of that time spent in REM. Overall you spend 75 percent of the night in Stages 1, 2, and 3, and 25 percent in REM. Your body knows what you need and adjusts the time in each stage accordingly.

For a good night's sleep, completing five sleep cycles is ideal, but you can get by on four.

To calculate the length of *your* sleep cycles, you do need a sleep tracker (go to page 46 for more info about devices). It will provide data about your passage through sleep stages. Measure the amount of time from one REM period to the next across four sleep cycles in a night. Tally that number and divide by four. Do this same process for seven nights, and then total your nightly averages, divide by seven, and get your weekly average of sleep cycle length.

> **Sleep Science:** If you regularly don't get enough sleep, your body compensates by spending more time in Stage 3 (deep sleep) and REM. Getting extra REM might seem like a dream come true, but it's not so much fun after all. You might experience a phenomenon called "REM rebound," with too-vivid dreams, nightmares, disorientation upon waking, and morning headaches.

WHAT ARE DREAMS?

In the broadest terms, dreams are mental movies, along with the sensations and feelings they evoke, that play on the underside of our eyelids mainly during REM. They might be in vivid color or black and white. They might distort time and space, or stick to normal, everyday dimensions. Rarely, people have lucid dreams when they are aware they are dreaming and can interact inside a dream with that knowledge.

Since dreams are produced by the mind, they reflect an individual's thoughts and experiences, although universal symbolism and themes do appear. If you can remember your dreams, you might be able to find some insight and meaning in them. Dreams about being stuck, teeth falling out, and showing up for a test without studying are common during stressful times. Dreams of flying, wealth, or fame might be wish fulfillment.

As for the "why" of dreams, science isn't 100 percent sure. Some believe dreams are like life's dress rehearsal, giving us a chance to play out scenarios—like having an affair—within the confines of our skulls. Regardless of whether your dreams make sense to you when you're awake, the brain produces them to help you sort through emotions and experiences from real life. Some research says that dreams are like "overnight therapy" that allows the brain to process painful life experiences.[13]

I consider dreams to be an emotional metabolism.

Some experiences might seem too painful to face while awake. The vast majority of PTSD sufferers—80 percent—have recurring nightmares, and the sleep anxiety and deprivation that go with them.

Dreams are thought to play a part in the memory consolidation process, although the "how" is murky. According to one hypothesis, our lives are kind of boring and routine and we need the weirdness of dreams to keep our minds sharp. But some dreams are themselves boring and routine, like one where you spend an hour cleaning the kitchen and going over to-do lists.

Sleep Myth: If you die in your dream, do you die in your sleep? (Is A Nightmare on Elm Street true?) Not too surprisingly, science has not attempted any studies of *inserting death dreams into people's heads and seeing whether they survive. Of course, people do die in their sleep from seizures, drug overdoses, and carbon monoxide poisoning. According to a 2021 study, 22 percent of all heart-related sudden deaths happen while sleeping.[14] Fifteen percent of ischemic strokes occur at night.[15] People with severe obstructive sleep apnea are three times as likely to die overnight than those who don't have it.[16] If you are in good health without risk factors (like a seizure disorder, heart or lung disease, obesity, or addiction), dying in your sleep is relatively rare. I wouldn't recommend watching a Freddy Krueger movie before bed, though. It might give you nightmares.*

CAN YOU DIE FROM NOT SLEEPING?

Several nights of insomnia might make you feel like a zombie.

Exhaustion-related irritability and mood swings might make your coworkers or partner secretly wish you dead. But there is no scientific evidence that acute sleep deprivation alone will kill a human being.

Sleep deprivation does affect lifestyle choices, mood, and cognition, in ways that are bad for you and those around you. When exhausted, you are

- less likely to exercise
- more likely to get injured while exercising[17]
- more likely to overeat and make unhealthy food choices[18]
- prone to anger[19]
- prone to go dark emotionally
- likely to struggle to regulate feelings[20]
- likely to suffer from cognitive impairment[21]

On top of how unmotivated, mean, sad, and, frankly, stupid we are when tired, chronic sleep deprivation can lead to developing such deadly diseases as diabetes[22] and cardiovascular disease.[23]

So when people joke, "I'll sleep when I'm dead," they can rest assured (or not) that their eternal slumber might come faster than they think.

So, yes, long-term sleep deprivation might indirectly do you in, and it'll certainly make you feel horrible until then.

Rats, on the other hand, are not so fortunate. In a 1989 University of Chicago study, researcher Allan Rechtschaffen subjected ten rats to an experiment. He put them on a platform in a tank full of water. And as soon as they started to fall asleep, the platform tilted and they fell into water, jolting them awake. Some of the rats died — or were euthanized upon imminent death — after eleven days of total sleep deprivation. The heartiest rodents survived without a wink for thirty-two days and were then put to sleep permanently.[24] As the experiment wore on, the rats grew lesions on their tails and paws. Their fur became discolored. They lost weight despite eating more. It wasn't pretty.

I wouldn't recommend experimenting with just how long you can last without sleep. But for science and/or glory, others have tried.

> **My Sleep Story**: *Our second child was born about eighteen months after our first. All new parents know that the sleep loss that first year is real — and it can take six years to pay off the sleep debt you rack up, according to a 2019 study[25] — but I think this story says it all: My wife had asked me to get the breast milk out of the fridge to make a bottle for our daughter. I was functioning on about three or four hours of sleep. I walked over to the linen closet, opened it up, and said to my wife, "Where is the f*cking milk, and why are there sheets in the fridge??"*

WHAT HAPPENS TO YOU IF YOU'RE SEVERELY SLEEP-DEPRIVED?

Californian Randy Gardner, age seventeen in December 1963, set out to break the record for going the longest without sleep. He stayed awake for eleven days and twenty-four minutes by playing pinball, table tennis, and basketball and by just remaining upright. To make sure he stayed awake in the bathroom, he had to keep talking to observers, including William Dement, PhD, MD, and founder of the Sleep Research Center at Stanford University, and Lieutenant Commander John J. Ross of the U.S. Navy Medical Neuropsychiatric Research Unit in San Diego. The doctors monitored Gardner's medical condition throughout.

After two days, Gardner got moody and couldn't do simple tongue twisters.

After four days, he started to hallucinate.

During days five, six, and seven, his speech slurred and he couldn't remember where he was or what he was doing.

By day eleven, he was non-responsive to questions and showed zero expressiveness.

Once he set a new record, Gardner went to sleep for fourteen hours straight and woke up refreshed, apparently unharmed. By multiple mental and physical measures, he was back to normal after just one good rest period.[26] Would that we all had the resilience of a healthy seventeen-year-old.

Gardner lived to tell the tale, and his experiment became fodder for scientific research on sleep deprivation for decades. But if he hadn't been so closely watched in a controlled setting, who knows what might have happened to him?

Even going **just one night without sleep** has a significant negative effect on brain function.[27] Expect symptoms such as brain fog, shortened attention span, crankiness, and a hair-trigger temper. Because it's harder to concentrate and make decisions while exhausted, you might not be able to complete simple tasks. Physically, your reaction time would be considerably slower. You might feel shaky and tense and yawn uncontrollably. Hearing and vision might fail.

According to a 2021 Ohio State University study, pulling an all-nighter causes cognitive impairment as profound as a concussion or a blood alcohol level of 0.10 percent (the legal limit to drive is 0.08 percent).[28] Speaking of which, drowsy driving is an accident — or a death — just waiting to happen. The National Highway Traffic Safety Administration estimates that 91,000 crashes were caused by drowsy drivers in 2017, resulting in 50,000 injuries and 800 deaths.[29] Why is drowsy driving so dangerous? Sleep deprivation means slower reflexes and reaction time. Any neurological performance deficit can be dangerous. One night of disrupted sleep makes it more likely you'll be killed crossing the street or kill someone else if you are behind the wheel.

My Sleep Story: Early in my career, I was working with the Georgia State Patrol. We were trying to discuss the similarities between drowsy driving and drunk driving. The officer I was speaking to told me a fact that I don't think I will ever forget. I asked him if he could tell the difference between a drowsy-driving and a drunk-driving accident, and he replied, "One hundred percent. I can tell just by walking up on the scene. With drowsy driving, there are never any skid marks because they are asleep and never hit the brakes. The crashes are usually more violent as well." Chilling.

Go **thirty-six hours without sleep** and your neurological impairment will get even worse. Along with having the attention span and focus of a fruit fly, you might have trouble coming up with the right word to describe something you can't remember anyway. Just getting off the couch will require a herculean effort. Your body will increase cortisol production, which triggers the "I'm under attack!" fight-or-flight sympathetic nervous system. You'll feel ravenous (like those poor tortured rats in Chicago) because a sleep-deprived body increases production of the "I'm starving" hormone ghrelin.[30] If you can't stop eating after a bad night's sleep, it's not your fault. It's ghrelin's.

After **forty-eight hours without sleep**, your brain might as well be pea soup. Your sense of reality will slip, leaving you with zero idea what's going on, including how hatefully and irritably you're behaving. Your immune system will be compromised. Defenses down, you become vulnerable to bacterial and viral illnesses.

Go **seventy-two hours without sleep** and your brain will kick into self-preservation mode, putting thoughts of lying down and closing your eyes on a loop. The only escape would be hallucinating, likely to happen at this point. Even the simplest tasks — doing basic math, writing an email, or making a sandwich — become difficult because you can't concentrate. Communication will be impossible due to slurred speech, paranoia, and even acute psychosis.[31]

Ninety-six hours without sleep could bring on a complete mental break from reality. The toxic buildup in the brain could cause it to malfunction. In a 2015 study in Taiwan, internal inflammation and oxidative stress related to prolonged sleep deprivation caused multiple organ failure in mice.[32] It'd take longer in humans, but any increased inflammation ups the risk for a host of diseases.

As I said, you might get bragging rights for being able to stay awake for days on end. You might get a Guinness World Records entry, like Minnesotan Zach Gensler, who played poker for 124 hours in 2021, pausing for just a few naps that Guinness required for safety reasons. But you won't be so cocky from a hospital bed.

HOW DO YOU KNOW IF YOU'RE GETTING ENOUGH QUALITY SLEEP?

Excellent question. And you'll find out in the next chapter.

TAKEAWAYS

- There's no absolute consensus about why we sleep, but we know that it is an essential, automatic function built into the human life cycle.
- The body is active during sleep, restoring and healing, forging neural pathways, and storing memories.
- Sleep drive is the mechanism that makes you progressively more tired as the day goes on.
- Sleep rhythm is your internal clock that tells you when to feel tired and when to wake up.
- The four sleep stages range from light to deep sleep, for recovery and rejuvenation, and the dreamy state of REM, for creativity and consolidation.
- A sleep cycle is all four stages of sleep, lasting approximately ninety minutes. You should have four or five cycles per night.
- You won't die from sleep deprivation, but if it's severe, you might wish you were dead.
- Chronic poor sleep affects cognition, attention, memory, and mood and disrupts bodily function.
- Prioritize quality sleep or put whole-body balance at risk.

CHAPTER 2

Sleep Assessment Tools

Before you can knock down the first Domino of Wellness
and sleep as if you were born to it (which you were),
start by assessing your sleep now.

SELF-REPORTED SLEEP DIARY

SELF-REPORTED QUALITY ASSESSMENT

SLEEP TRACKERS

To improve at anything, it's best to have metrics to measure your progress. Get a baseline and strive to improve from there. In this chapter, you're going to collect some data and establish baselines on two sleep factors: quantity (duration) and quality (depth).

Together, quantity and quality paint a pretty good picture of how well—or how poorly—you sleep. They both matter. Quite often, patients come to me and say, "I don't know what's going on. I sleep for eight or nine hours a night, and I'm still exhausted each morning." This sounds a lot like "I go to the gym and do cardio for hours but still don't feel fit." Minimal testing is required to reveal that, although they are down for many hours, their sleep skims the surface because of sleep apnea, alcohol consumption, smoking, or medications that disrupt deep sleep. If you spend most of the night in Stages 1 and 2, you won't reap the restorative benefits of Stage 3 or REM—and wake up exhausted.

The reverse might also be true. Some of my patients successfully pass through each stage and have efficient, quality sleep; they just don't get nearly enough of it to function optimally.

HOW LONG DO YOU NEED TO SLEEP?

Everyone is different, and we have different sleep needs based on factors such as fitness level, medications, lifestyle, and chronotype (genetically predetermined preference for morning or evening activity; read all about chronotypes in my previous book *The Power of When*). A crucial factor is how old you are. According to the National Sleep Foundation, sleep need differs widely by age group.[1]

- Newborns (up to four months): 14–17 hours of sleep per twenty-four hours
- Infants (four to eleven months): 12–15 hours
- Toddlers (one to two years): 11–14 hours

- Preschoolers (three to five years): 10–13 hours
- School-age children (six to twelve): 9–11 hours
- Teens (twelve to eighteen): 8–10 hours
- Young adults (nineteen to twenty-five): 7–9 hours
- Adults (twenty-five to sixty-four): 7–9 hours
- Advanced adults (over sixty-five): 7–8 hours

To calculate sleep need for most of the adult population, use a basic formula. Most people function at their best if they log five complete sleep cycles. Sleep cycles vary in length depending on the individual and the time of night, ranging from 50 to 120 minutes. But 90 minutes is a useful average.

5 x 90 = 450 minutes or 7.5 hours

Sleep Science: *Eight hours is a myth. The math does not even work. When we look at the "recommended amount of sleep," we can go back to the preindustrial age, when people kept a biphasic sleep schedule, taking "first sleep" from 9:00 p.m. to midnight, then awakening to do things like eat, have sex, and pray, then taking a "second sleep" from 2:00 a.m. until dawn. These two phases made up seven or eight hours of sleep. After the industrial revolution came along and we could work at night, sleep got compacted into a single, longer stretch.*

So how can you figure out if you get enough sleep? Wearable sleep trackers like smartwatches, straps, and rings can provide data on multiple sleep parameters. But so can a no-tech method I recommend to all my patients: **a sleep diary**.

Not only is self-reported information valid, the process of proactively writing things down gets people invested in sleep improvement as an obtainable goal. By recording data like a scientist, some people can detach emotionally from their sleep issues, which goes a long way to reducing anxiety about it. (That said, for others, keeping an accurate record can produce anxiety and exacerbate insomnia.) By taking a few minutes to fill in the information, ideally at the same time every day, you also create a habit of self-care. The drawback of keeping a sleep diary is diminished accuracy. You might know the specific minute you get in bed, but it's hard to say exactly when you fell asleep. Bear in mind that the sleep diary worked well enough for about twenty-five years before we had anything else.

SLEEP DIARY							
	M	T	W	Th	F	S	Su
I went to bed at...							
I fell asleep at...							
I woke up ____ times in the night...							
I woke up at...							
I snoozed the alarm ____ times...							
I got out of bed at...							
I had ____ caffeinated drinks...							
I had ____ alcoholic drinks...							
I napped for...							
I exercised for...							

Self-Reported Sleep Diary

You can design a sleep diary with pen and paper, create a spreadsheet, or download the template I use with my patients.* The simplest version is on the previous page.

The point of the diary is to chart averages and notice trends, not just in how long and well you sleep, but how other factors affect your sleep. If you keep a diary for even three days, you will be able to see how exercise and alcohol affect sleep onset (falling asleep) and sleep maintenance (staying asleep), and you can then adjust your behavior.

After keeping a sleep diary for seven days, add the total number of hours you slept and divide that number by seven to get an average.

On average, how many hours did you sleep per night?

_____

Was the number different on weekend days?

_____

What time did you usually get up?

_____

Was the time different on weekend days?

_____

Many of my patients end up taking the sleep diary, re-creating it digitally, and just punching in numbers on a keyboard. That's more convenient, I suppose. But let me tell you, every time I insist that people write things down with a pen on paper, sleep improvement comes faster and is more profound. Clinically speaking, I don't

---

* Go to drive.google.com/file/d/1Nd21vH5RNNem8s73ga228khxRCfEj7Iq /view

know why the act of handwriting a sleep diary makes the healing process more effective. I just know that it does. Perhaps, by writing it down directly, patients understand the importance of the process, are closer to insight about what the data means, and see the trends more clearly.

HOW WELL DO YOU SLEEP?

We tend to focus on sleep quantity over quality. I can't tell you how many people have asked me, "How much sleep do I *really* need?" (See above; roughly seven and a half hours per night.) Everyone seems to focus on minutes or hours, but if the sleep is not good quality, the amount of time doesn't matter.

Sleep quality is as important for overall health and wellness as quantity is.

Because we live in a 24/7 culture with constant stimulation and environmental factors that disrupt sleep (artificial light, noise, screens), not to mention use of substances that hinder sleep (caffeine, tobacco, alcohol, cannabis, and medications such as antidepressants), our society is in a sleep quality crisis. Light from devices pouring into our eyes in the dark hours has been proven time and again to interfere with circadian rhythm and REM quality.[2] Subpar REM quality keeps the brain from being able to learn, memorize, restore, and refresh. Not ideal for the world we live in, where things move at fiberoptic speed.

Measuring how well one sleeps is harder than doing basic math. A significant *quality* factor is spending sufficient time in each sleep stage to reap all the restorative potential from light sleep, deep sleep, and REM. The other quality factor that makes assessment a challenge is knowing how many times you wake up during the night. You *might* be able to keep track of wake-ups, but sleep stages? That information is not accessible on your own.

If you went to a sleep lab for an overnight assessment and were hooked up to twenty-seven electrodes, you would get very accurate diagnostics about sleep quality, but the environment (sleeping in a strange place, having wires attached to you) may make the findings inaccurate. At sleepdoctor.com, we sell an at-home version called a WatchPAT ONE kit, which includes finger, wrist, and chest sensors, for under $200. It's not as sophisticated as sleep lab equipment, but it's more accurate than the wearable sleep-tracking devices generally available to the public. And you could also consider a wearable sleep tracker; however, be careful: Many do not have accurate measurements and use differing definitions. (I review trackers, what I use them for, and which ones I like, on page 46.)

But honestly, you don't have to buy a device to get a decent sense of how well you're sleeping. Just do a self-reported quality assessment. I like to focus a self-reported assessment on getting what I call a "morning feel" statistic. One top priority for most people is to wake up feeling positive, so let's see how that changes as you change some of your sleep behaviors!

Self-Reported Quality Assessment

The standard assessment tool for sleep quality is the Pittsburgh Sleep Quality Index, developed in 1989 by researchers at the University of Pittsburgh.[3] I've shortened and adapted it into a multiple-choice quiz for simplicity and ease of scoring.

Quiz: How Well Are You Sleeping?

Give the most accurate answers for the following statements.

During the past month:

1. I feel refreshed when I wake up in the morning.

   a. Always

   b. Sometimes

   c. Rarely

2. I feel satisfied with the sleep I'm getting.

    a. Always

    b. Sometimes

    c. Rarely

3. The overall quality of my sleep is:

    a. Good

    b. Okay

    c. Not great

4. I take a medication to help me sleep.

    a. Less than once a week

    b. Up to twice a week

    c. Three or more times a week

5. I lie awake for at least thirty minutes before I fall asleep.

    a. Less than once a week

    b. Up to twice a week

    c. Three or more times a week

6. I wake up in the middle of the night or very early in the morning and can't fall back asleep.

    a. Less than once a week

    b. Up to twice a week

    c. Three or more times a week

7. I get up to use the bathroom during the night.

    a. Less than once a week

    b. Up to twice a week

    c. Three or more times a week

8. I cough a lot at night or snore loudly.

    a. Less than once a week

    b. Up to twice a week

    c. Three or more times a week

9. My bedroom feels too cold or too hot.

    a. Less than once a week

    b. Up to twice a week

    c. Three or more times a week

10. I have bad dreams.

    a. Less than once a week

    b. Up to twice a week

    c. Three or more times a week

11. I have pain that keeps me from sleeping.

    a. Less than once a week

    b. Up to twice a week

    c. Three or more times a week

12. If I sleep with a partner, they snore or otherwise interrupt my sleep.

    a. Less than once a week

    b. Up to twice a week

    c. Three or more times a week

13. During the day, I lack enthusiasm about getting things done.

    a. Less than once a week

    b. Up to twice a week

    c. Three or more times a week

14. During the day, I have trouble staying awake during normal activity.

    a. Less than once a week

    b. Up to twice a week

    c. Three or more times a week

15. During the day, I have anxiety about whether I'll get enough sleep that night.

    a. Less than once a week

    b. Up to twice a week

    c. Three or more times a week

SELF-REPORTED SLEEP QUALITY ASSESSMENT SCORING

This quiz assesses sleep quality in a few different ways: subjective satisfaction, disruptions, and efficiency.

Satisfaction: For statements 1 through 4, give yourself 2 points for (a) answers, 1 point for (b) answers, and 0 points for (c) answers. **Total points:** _____

  0 to 3: You are deeply unsatisfied with the quality of your sleep.

  4 to 6: You are somewhat satisfied with the quality of your sleep.

  7 to 8: You are highly satisfied with the quality of your sleep.

Disruptions: For statements 5 through 12, give yourself 2 points for (a) answers, 1 point for (b) answers, and 0 points for (c) answers. **Total points:** _____

  0 to 5: Your sleep is often disrupted, a good reason for a likely low satisfaction score.

  6 to 10: Your sleep is sometimes disrupted.

  11 to 16: Your sleep is rarely disrupted—lucky you!

Efficiency: For statements 13 through 15, give yourself 2 points for (a) answers, 1 point for (b) answers, and 0 points for (c) answers. **Total points:** _____

0 to 2: Your sleep is inefficient rest and restoration to get you through the day.

3 to 4: Your sleep is somewhat efficient.

5 to 6: Your sleep is highly efficient.

Data on sleep quality is useful if it points to problem areas, and this quiz certainly gives you some clues about why you might have unsatisfying, low-quality, inefficient sleep. As you make changes to your routine, you'll see those numbers rise.

Sleep Science: Not all morning drowsiness means you've had insufficient or low-quality sleep. Feeling confused, almost drunk, and disoriented upon waking might be due to the phenomenon called "sleep inertia." It's the unfortunate result of your alarm going off while you're in deep, Delta-wave sleep. If this is a chronic occurrence, you might have a sleep disorder and should get some testing.[4] You may also be waking up out of sync with your chronotype's natural rhythm; we will get to that later.

THE HIGH-TECH APPROACH
SLEEP TRACKERS

I've given you no-tech methods for assessing sleep quantity and quality. But we live in the digital age. Most of us are walking around with smartphones or smartwatches/rings, many of which have apps that track sleep. I have to say that accuracy on such devices is not great, especially when it comes to tracking sleep onset and sleep stages.

Devices provide a lot of information, and checking your score each morning is fun. But don't freak out if your stats are horrible.

The watch strap might have been loose, or the battery ran out of juice, or the software is glitchy. Devices are never going to be as reliable as the diagnostic equipment at a sleep lab. They are no more reliable than no-tech methods.[5] But if you are curious about tracking sleep with technology, I have some recommendations.

Wearables. The promise is that you can strap on wellness! Good sleep is only as far away as your wrist! Or finger! Or forehead! Again, take all the data with a grain of salt. Here are the pros and cons of four popular devices:

Whoop Strap

Cost: $240, includes a one-year membership

Pros: The strap device is comfortable and minimally invasive when exercising or sleeping. It's not particularly attractive, but it's okay. It has many sensors for measuring heart rate, blood oxygen, respiratory rate, skin temperature, and movement. All that data yields accurate data on sleep onset, wake-ups, and sleep stages. It's also got an alarm that wakes you up with gentle vibrations. Battery life: four to five days!

Cons: You must become a member to use it.

Oura Ring

Cost: $350 starting price, plus $6 monthly fee

Pros: This is the one I use and recommend to all my patients. It's very attractive, with several finishes to choose from (black, gold, rose gold, silver, etc.). It's comfortable, and unobtrusive. The sensors track temperature, blood oxygen, pulse, movement, and heart rate variability ... so, basically everything you need. You get daily reminders about bedtimes, based on daily activity and sleep history. Battery life: seven days!

Cons: You have to pay a monthly fee.

Muse S Headband

Cost: $400, plus a $12 per month premium subscription

Pros: Its sensors use EEG technology to track brain waves, providing the most accurate data on sleep quality, intensity, and quantity. It also tracks your sleep position — which can provide fascinating insight — and heart rate, too.

Cons: You wear it on your head, so it's not as comfortable as a wrist device or ring. You need a Bluetooth connection to use it, and you must charge it daily. It's *pricey*! Battery life: ten hours.

Apollo Neuro

Cost: $350, plus $99 membership

Pros: Versatility. You can wear this device on a wrist or ankle strap or clip it to your shirt, as long as it touches your skin. The tech uses low-intensity vibrations in certain patterns that either trigger the parasympathetic nervous system to put you into calm mode or activate the sympathetic nervous system to make you more alert. So you program the device to calm you down as needed, making it a sleep aid as much as a sleep tracker that collects data on all the sleep quantity, quality, and movement. It's comfortable to wear, and not unattractive.

Cons: You have to program it on your phone app. Battery life: six to eight hours.

> ***Sleep Science***: *So many people come up to me and say, "Tonight I had a good night's sleep. Then I woke up and looked at my tracker score. It told me I had a bad night – ? The opposite is true, too. I had a horrible night and woke up to find a decent score? What gives?" Or someone says, "Dr. Breus, I only got fourteen minutes of deep sleep. Is that okay?" Here is the thing about looking at each stage, each*

cycle, and all that data. If you don't know what it means, it could be confusing and downright frustrating. More importantly, no one should look at their data every day. It's simply too small a sample to draw any conclusions. I advise everyone to look at trends in their data over a week or a month and to use the information to make your own calculations about, say, the length of your sleep cycles (I showed you how on page 27) and the right bedtime for you (I'll show you how on page 83).

After keeping a sleep diary and doing a quality assessment, or wearing a tracker for a few days, you'll have a sense of whether you are getting enough, and good enough, sleep. If you are among the sleep-deprived or sleep-deficient third of Americans, your logical next question is, "So what am I doing wrong?"

I got you. Just turn the page.

TAKEAWAYS

- Sleep quantity — how many hours of sleep you need — varies depending on age and other factors.
- Keeping a diary of your sleep habits can help determine the right sleep quantity for you.
- Quality sleep is getting sufficient time in each sleep stage for overall restoration.
- Wearable trackers are great tools for assessment. I still recommend keeping a handwritten sleep diary, which is as effective as a high-tech device.

CHAPTER 3

Troubleshooting Sleep

*The consequences of poor sleep make an exhaustive list.
And the reasons people don't get enough sleep
are all too common and often self-inflicted.*

THE CONSEQUENCES

compromised immunity
increased inflammation
low energy
weight issues
mental health problems
emotional regulation issues
shorter lifespan

THE TOP FIVE SLEEP TRAPS

living out of sync with your circadian rhythm
playing catch-up
freaking out
sleep-disrupting habits
hoping the problem goes away on its own

Before I get into some of the most common and easiest-to-fix sleep challenges, let's talk about what's really at stake if you don't get adequate and efficient sleep each night. It's a frightening list. I'm not trying to scare you or pile on pressure and anxiety, but as they say, sometimes the truth hurts! I choose sleep as the first domino that needs to be knocked down because of how consequential it is to overall wellness.

On top of feeling exhausted—and the cognitive and personality problems that go along with that—bad sleepers can expect to deal with these medical and psychological issues:

Compromised immunity. Your body's white blood cells rush to infection sites to kill off foreign intruders such as bacteria and viruses. These foot soldiers of immunity are always on the hunt for free radicals (rogue cells that cause inflammation and, in some cases, tumors) to neutralize them. When your body is in balance, white blood cell production and motility is robust. Immunity cells get where they need to go and do the job they are supposed to do. But on little sleep, your immune system falls into chaos. White blood cells can't get where they need to go to fight infection.

Carnegie Mellon University did a study on sleep and immunity with 153 healthy adults between twenty-one and fifty-five. For fourteen consecutive days, the subjects self-reported how long and how well they slept and whether they felt rested. Then they were quarantined in a lab and given nasal drops that contained common-cold germs. The subjects who slept for seven hours a night on average were three times more likely to be coughing and sneezing than those who slept for eight hours. Just one hour made the difference between getting sick and staying well.[1] Per a 2017 UCLA study, if you sleep for four hours *for just one night*, the motility of "natural killer cells" (immunity cells that fight cancer, among other jobs) can be reduced by up to 72 percent.[2] Other studies link short sleep with a greater risk for diabetes,[3] high blood pressure,[4] cardiovascular disease, and obesity.

50

Increased inflammation. For a 2020 study published in *Frontiers in Neurology*, 533 subjects kept sleep diaries, submitted to actigraphy testing in sleep labs, and gave blood samples to track their inflammatory biomarkers. Over seven nights, operational sleep inconsistencies—wake-ups, variations in bedtimes and wake times, etc.—were measured. These disruptions were associated with higher levels of inflammatory biomarkers, at least in women.[5]

Low energy. I've already explained how the buildup of adenosine increases throughout the day, making you more tired. Sleep clears away that chemical, helping you feel clean-slate fresh and energized in the morning. Glycogen, stored glucose that fuels the body to do pretty much everything, has the opposite relationship with sleep. During rest, glycogen goes up, preparing the body for an energized day. But if you're sleep-deprived, your body's stores of this quick energy source decrease, leaving you dragging.[6] Certain behaviors, such as eating nutrient-dense whole foods and exercising, give people more energy. A diet lacking in vitamins, minerals, and protein makes you feel sluggish *and* interferes with sleep. Same thing with not moving enough.[7] If you're too tired from short sleep to eat well or exercise, you won't enjoy the energy—or quality sleep the following night—that a healthy diet and movement can bring.

A Patient's Sleep Story: A patient of mine was hit hard after being downsized. The circumstantial frustration and anxiety brought about insomnia symptoms that she'd never experienced before. She didn't connect her sleep deprivation with feeling too low energy to meet a friend for lunch or update her résumé. She'd had sleepless nights before, and never experienced this. The one-two punch of a trying emotional time mixed with fewer hours of sleep did her in. She got in a pattern of not sleeping or exercising. Suddenly, any small task felt overwhelming. I got her on a sleep reset plan – which you will be doing in the Sleep-Drink-Breathe Plan later on – and she recovered her normal energy levels … and got a new job.

Weight issues. New term alert that I just made up: "Tunger" is eating because you're tired. It's real. It makes you put on weight. For a 2014 Brigham Young study of 330 college-age women, scientists monitored their sleep patterns over a seven-day period, along with height, weight, and body-fat percentage. There was a clear association between the subjects who cycled through all four sleep stages at least five times per night (sleep efficiency), keeping set bedtime and wake time (sleep consistency), and having a normal weight with a lower body-fat percentage. Those with low sleep efficiency and consistency tended to be overweight.[8]

For a National Institutes of Health study, researchers tracked the sleep habits and body mass indexes (BMIs) of 496 adults for over a decade. After factoring in family history, demographics, and exercise habits, they found that the subjects who slept less were significantly more likely to be obese.[9] Lack of sleep has long been associated with increases in ghrelin, the hunger hormone, and decreases in leptin, the satiety hormone.[10] The thickness of one's neck and/or midsection predicts for obstructive sleep apnea (OSA), a life-threatening disorder that lowers the quality and quantity of sleep. Which came first, being overweight or having OSA? It doesn't matter. Having excess pounds can make it harder to sleep; not sleeping makes you gain weight. (My book *The Sleep Doctor's Diet Plan: Simple Rules for Losing Weight While You Sleep* goes into this in depth, if you'd like to read more.)

Mental health issues. Even a little sleep insufficiency fogs your mind and wrecks focus, concentration, and response time. You're more likely to make terrible decisions that you regret later when tired.[11] And your risk of depression[12] and anxiety disorder goes through the roof. There is a bidirectional relationship between poor sleep and anxiety, meaning each one causes the other. If you lie awake at night, ruminating anxiously about how you're not sleeping, you're more likely to get depressed, too.[13]

A Patient's Sleep Story: Anxiety causes sleep issues, which amp up anxiety, and so on: It's a vicious circle that keeps getting smaller, shrinking people's lives. One man in his twenties came to me because, as he said, "My entire life is about worrying whether I'll sleep, not sleeping, and then worrying again the next day. I've been reduced to being that guy, the one who drags himself around, begs off doing anything, and says stupid things because I'm too tired to be smart." To break the cycle, I worked with him on acceptance first. If he doesn't sleep, it's okay. Relieving the pressure to accomplish sleep lowered his anxiety just enough to drift off. More sleep meant less anxiety, and before long, both his sleep and outlook improved.

Emotional regulation problems. Poor sleep makes it harder for people to cope with the stressors of everyday life. Even with the Calm app playing in your ears nonstop, it's difficult to regulate intense emotions when exhausted. Although sleep experts have empirical data that proves daytime emotional stress affects dream content and how you feel within a dream, the exact mechanisms are not yet clear. However, according to 2017 research, if you feel stressed all day and manage to fall asleep at night, REM sleep — when you should be consolidating memory, processing life events and emotions — is delayed and disrupted by wake-ups.[14]

In other words,
if you're burned out and overwhelmed,
sleep isn't going to make it all better.

For a 2020 Australian study of some 326 young adults, subjects were tested with actigraphy and self-reported their sleep duration, efficiency, disruptions, and quality over a week. Also, during that time, they reported on their stress levels in the morning, afternoon, and evening. The subjects who complained of stress in the evening had short sleep the night before. Short, disrupted sleep predicted for high stress the next day.[15] It never fails. Bad sleep → stress → bad sleep → stress, on and on in a loop from hell.

Shorter lifespan. Middle-aged and early-old-age poor sleepers might be shaving years off their lives. Per 2020 research, a 5 percent decrease in REM sleep starting in your fifties has been associated with a 13 percent greater risk of all-cause mortality (dying for any reason) within twenty years.[16] So if you are losing sleep to work hard and bank as much money as possible before retirement age, you might never get to enjoy it.

⁛

Of course, everyone knows intuitively that good sleep brings good health. If you can just get enough, and good enough, sleep, you'll be healthier, slimmer, and less stressed, anxious, and depressed. It *is* that simple.

But life is complicated. Sometimes the way we live doesn't line up with getting a good night's sleep night after night. Bad habits and misinformation are what you're up against in the pursuit of knocking down this all-important domino.

In my decades as a practicing sleep doctor, I've isolated the **Top Five Sleep Traps** that rob people of consistently logging a good night's rest. How many sleep blunders are you making?

SLEEP TRAP #1: LIVING OUT OF SYNC
WITH YOUR CIRCADIAN RHYTHM

Your body comes preinstalled with a biological clock, a circadian rhythm or chronorhythm. Your chronorhythm encompasses *dozens* of internal clocks that tell you when to do everything—sleep, wake, eat, digest, think, imagine, have sex, feel social, among hundreds of other functions. The timing of your circadian rhythms is an important clue to your chronotype—your genetic predisposition for being an early riser or a late riser or falling somewhere in between. There truly is a best time to do just about everything, as long as you know your chronotype.*

In my research working with thousands of patients, I've identified four distinct chronotypes with hormonal ebbs and flows, personalities, and lifestyles that are unique to each. To discover your chronotype, go to chronoquiz.com. Over two million people have taken the short quiz. Having this personal insight can be life changing, especially for sleep issues.

Briefly, the four chronotypes are:

Bears. Bears, like their animal counterparts, are diurnal, meaning they are active in the daytime and restful at night. They account for 50 percent of the general population. Since they have the majority, society's time has been built around their schedule. For example, the 9-to-5 workday was designed for Bears, who rise naturally around 7:00 a.m. and start to lose their cognitive sharpness in the later afternoon. Not to say that they spring out of bed. Rising is a process for them of hitting the snooze button and dragging themselves up. (If they could, they'd hibernate all winter.) Their peak energy hours are mid-morning to mid-afternoon and

---

* My book *The Power of When* is all about chronorhythms and chronotypes. If you want to go deeper on this fascinating subject, you can pick up a copy wherever books are sold.

then early evening (happy hour), when they get a second wind. Their tired hours are late afternoon around 3:00 p.m. and bedtime around 11:00 p.m. Bears are often extroverts, but I have met plenty of introvert Bears as well. They love food and would gladly graze all day. Exercise-wise, they tend to be weekend warriors who enjoy team sports with friends. Even-keel Bears are conflict averse in relationships and have predictable mood shifts based on life circumstances.

Lions. Like their animal counterparts, human Lions are pre-dawn hunters, waking up hungry and full of energy. They account for 20 percent of the general population. Although many people have "Lion envy," wishing they were natural early risers—Lions' eyes snap open before dawn. Their energy stays high until about 5:00 p.m., when it starts to rapidly decline, landing them in bed by 9:00 or 10:00 p.m. It's hard, if not impossible, for them to go to parties and social events at night. Lions are health conscious, exercising regularly, eating well, and avoiding drugs and alcohol. Of all the chronotypes, they have the lowest BMI. They are ambitious, born leaders, fearless, goal oriented, confident, and optimistic. Cognitively, peak clarity hits in the early morning, when most of the world is just waking up.

Wolves. Wolves in nature are nocturnal, coming alive when the rest of the world goes to sleep. Their human equivalents account for about 20 percent of the general population. This chronotype doesn't feel tired until midnight or later. Mornings pass by in a fog. They might appear awake, making coffee, getting dressed, making more coffee, but their brains are still half asleep. By the afternoon, when their minds finally clear, Wolves are ravenous. They tend to eat most of their calories later in the day, which is one of the reasons their BMI is higher than the other chronotypes'. Pleasure seekers, Wolves indulge their impulses, desires, and appetites. They'd rather go to the bar than the gym. Their concentration peaks in the afternoon, when they can finally focus enough to write a chapter of their novel. Although they love to party, Wolves need a lot of alone time, too.

Dolphins. In nature, dolphins are unihemispheric sleepers. Half their brain is awake to prevent drowning and watch for predators while the other half sleeps. Human Dolphins are insomniacs who never seem to fall into deep, sustained sleep. Just 10 percent of the population, Dolphins' hormonal cycles are the upside-down version of Bears', Lions', and Wolves'. For example, when the others' cortisol drops at night, Dolphins' secretions go up. They tend to be neurotic and risk averse, so they avoid harmful substances and stick with doctor-approved healthy habits. They have below-average BMIs, due to obsessive exercise and fidgeting. Dolphins are loyal and loving partners, but their neuroticism can be a bit much for the average Bear. At work, super-smart Dolphins are detail oriented, with high standards, peaking creatively mid-morning. They struggle with winding down before bed and get anxious about their habitual sleep issues.

Which chronotype are you? _____

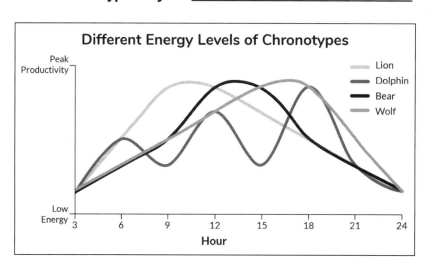

If chronorhythms were the only factor, Bears would have the easiest time getting adequate quality sleep. After all, conventional scheduling—rise at seven, lunch at noon, dinner at six, bedtime at eleven—was designed by and for them. The other half of the population is forced to stick to conventional eating, working, and sleeping schedules that force them to live out of sync with their natural rhythm, causing profound issues, most notably with sleep.

A Wolf patient of mine was convinced she'd been struggling with severe insomnia her whole life. But when she learned that she was an extreme Wolf and was going to bed before her body was ready for sleep, her whole life changed. Her "sleeper" was not broken. She was a Wolf trying to cram her life into a Bear's schedule. I said, "Don't get in bed until 1:00 a.m." As an empty-nest freelancer, she could adjust her schedule accordingly. Suddenly, she fell asleep within fifteen minutes of her head hitting the pillow. A lifetime of frustration was gone. She set her alarm for 9:00 a.m. instead of seven, but she didn't need it. Her body woke her up naturally at 8:45 a.m.

"It's like my body had a built-in alarm clock," she said.

It does. And so does yours. You might not know what it is.

Bears' inner alarms are set for around 7:30 a.m. But if they stay up late, their circadian rhythm gets mixed up and readjusts itself based on behavior—a phenomenon called "social jet lag." Even though society runs on Bear time, they don't necessarily stick with the schedule. And that leads to sleep deprivation because they still have to wake up at a certain time to meet the demands of the day.

Lions' inner alarm goes off at 6:00 a.m. or earlier. Even if they force themselves to stay up way past their genetically preferred bedtime, they will still bolt up at or before dawn.

Dolphins struggle to fall asleep because they are alert and energized when conventional timing would have them get in bed and close their eyes. They wind up staring at the ceiling for hours, anxiety building, until they nod off and get four sleep cycles if they're lucky.

CHRONOTYPES' IDEAL WAKE AND BEDTIMES
Set an alarm on your phone!

If each chronotype knew—and stuck to—their genetically preferred bed- and wake times, they'd be more successful sleepers. It might not always be possible, but the closer you can get to living in sync with your chronorhythm, the better off you'll be.

Cortisol is the guide here. It stops flowing at night to calm you down and is released in the early morning to wake you up. After one to two hours of cortisol increase, your body is ready to begin the day. According to a study of serum blood levels,[17] the average (Bear) morning cortisol increase starts between 5:00 and 6:00 a.m. Scale that metric one or two hours earlier for Lions, and one to two hours later for Wolves.

Bears should wake around 7:30 a.m. and get in bed around 11:00 p.m., giving them a thirty-minute buffer to fall sleep, netting them eight hours per night.

Lions will wake up at 6:00 a.m. If they can stay awake until 10:00 p.m., they will get their five cycles easily. Extreme Lions can shift this to a 5-to-9 wake-sleep schedule.

Wolves should not even look at a bed until midnight, and if possible, wake no earlier than 8:00 a.m. Moving closer to this schedule can net Wolves more time sleeping, rather than lying fully awake, wondering anxiously when sleep is going to happen.

Dolphins, as always, are a special case. Their cortisol, body temperature, and blood pressure are elevated throughout the night and drop in the morning. They are just not made for deep, continuous sleep. But if they rise at 7:00 a.m., they can build up enough sleep drive to fall asleep by 1:00 a.m. and get a sufficient six hours of rest.

> **Sleep Shortcut**: *Of special note: If you must choose only one, either bedtime or wake time, I suggest you make your wake-up time consistent. First, it probably already is, at least five days a week, and second, the morning wake-up is the anchor of good sleep. If all you ever did was wake up based on your chronotype, your sleep would improve dramatically!*

SLEEP TRAP #2: PLAYING CATCH-UP

Most people know that insufficient sleep is terrible for their physical, mental, and emotional health and well-being. They try to get seven or eight hours per night, the recommended amount for adults and seniors. But that doesn't seem to work. TikTok is not going to scroll itself until midnight, after all. When people fail to get the golden 450 minutes per night and start to rack up serious sleep debt, they think, "It's okay. I'll make up for it on the weekend."

The simple fact is, getting more sleep over one or two days per week doesn't mitigate the long-term detrimental effects of chronic sleep deprivation. It's like saying that you can lose weight by eating only salad on Saturday and Sunday. Or you can cure smoking-related lung damage by quitting cigarettes on the weekends.

The math does not add up. Say you get an average of six hours of sleep instead of 7.5 per weekday night. Your sleep debt calculation would be 5 (days) x 1.5 (hours of insufficient sleep per night) = 7.5 hours. If you attempted to pay back that debt on Saturday and Sunday, you'd need to sleep an additional 3.25 hours—or a continuous 10.75 hours—per night. I have not met many healthy adults who can sleep for nearly eleven hours straight, much less do it twice in a row.

My advice is to limit sleeping in on the weekend to forty-five extra minutes only. That can buy you back 1.5 hours of sleep per week, a dent in your debt. Why so strict about this? Oversleeping on the weekends sets up the phenomenon called "Sunday night insomnia," also called "social jet lag." Because you slept so late on Sunday morning, your sleep rhythm thinks you've moved to a different time zone and are on a new time schedule. So when you get in bed on Sunday night, you wind up lying awake for hours, leaving you exhausted Monday morning. It can take days to undo the circadian reset of sleeping late on the weekends. By Wednesday or Thursday, you will be back to the schedule for your time zone, but you'll have accrued hours of sleep debt.

> **Sleep Suggestion**: *Instead of catching up on sleep on the weekend and setting yourself up for a miserable week ahead, use Saturday and Sunday to get back on your natural chronorhythm. And stick to your ideal bed- and wake times. That way, you'll stack the sleep deck in your favor for the upcoming week and might slowly pay down long-overdue sleep debt.*

TOO MUCH: NOT A GOOD THING

Not to sound like Goldilocks, but getting too much sleep, or oversleeping, isn't ideal. Some people need nine hours to feel like themselves, or maybe you're recovering from an illness, making up for lost sleep, or you just had an emotionally or physically exhausting day. Oversleeping in those cases is fine, even good for you. But if you stay down for longer than eight hours regularly, and still wake up feeling tired, have a tough time waking and getting up, feel groggy throughout the day, and have trouble concentrating and remembering things, you might have a problem. Some potential explanations are depression, low sleep quality, and a sleep disorder such as narcolepsy, obstructive sleep apnea, or a circadian rhythm issue.

If oversleeping is chronic (more than three months), it's possible you have a sleep disorder called hypersomnia, characterized by feeling tired all the time despite long sleeping. Some hypersomnia causes are a head injury, stroke, Parkinson's disease, depression, bipolar disorder, and seasonal affective disorder. The risk factors are, ironically, similar to those of sleep deprivation, including diabetes, obesity, and cardiovascular disease.[18] It's not that oversleep causes these conditions; it's just associated with them.

If you are a parent and notice that your teen is oversleeping or you're a young adult who can't get out of bed, take this seriously. It could be a sign of depression. Forty percent of people under thirty have hypersomnia.[19] But oversleep is associated with depression in older people, too. In a 2018 study, among the depressed subjects, 30 percent experienced insomnia *and* hypersomnia.[20] They couldn't fall asleep and couldn't get out of bed.

The first step to getting to the bottom of why you might be oversleeping is to visit your doctor and do some testing for underlying conditions; also check your medications as a possible cause. Next, follow the recommendations in this book about setting consistent wake and bedtimes and avoiding alcohol, caffeine, nicotine, intense exercise, and exposure to electronics before bed. Add exercise earlier in the day so that you'll be able to fall asleep at the set time and enjoy quality rest that makes it easier to get out of bed in the morning.

SLEEP TRAP #3: FREAKING OUT

At the end of a sleep cycle, it's very common to wake up for a short while—a few seconds or a couple of minutes—before falling back into light sleep and beginning a new cycle. However, for people with sleep maintenance insomnia, those middle-of-the-night wake-ups can last so long that they cut into overall sleep duration. You might be in bed for eight hours, but unconscious for less than seven. That small but significant difference can tip the scales into sleep insufficiency.

The first thing most of us do when we wake up long enough to realize we're not immediately drifting off again is to look at a clock or check your phone to see what time it is. Next, you start doing mental math, as in, "It's three in the morning. That means I have four hours before I have to get up." Anxiety amps up, and you give yourself demands and warnings like "Go back to sleep RIGHT NOW. This instant! If you don't, you'll be a wreck all day tomorrow."

With anxiety comes cortisol and an accelerated heart rate and blood pressure, the physiological conditions that signal to the brain that it's time to rise, despite the dark hour.

If you're full of anxiety about not sleeping, your heart rate could jump to 100 beats per minute (BPM) just lying there. A healthy resting heart rate for adults is between 60 and 100 BPM. To reenter a sleep state, your heart rate should be 10 to 20 percent lower than that. So if your typical resting heart rate is 60, your sleep onset rate would be 48 to 54. If your resting heart rate is 80, your sleep onset rate would be 64 to 72. If you get up to use the bathroom, your heart rate will increase because of the activity, and it'll take even more time to slow down again.

If you can avoid it, don't get up to pee. Don't turn on the light, read, or walk aimlessly around the house. For the love of God, *do not look at your phone or any screen* and start doomscrolling. It'll send melatonin-suppressing blue light into your eyes, and it'll engage and excite your mind.

Instead, have a quick sip of water and just lie back down. Mentally reframe wakefulness as nonsleep deep rest. Being still, quiet, and at peace is still rejuvenating on some level. And in this state, you're more likely to drift back into actual sleep than if you were more physically or mentally active and stressed.

I tell patients, "Sleep is like love. The less you look for it, the more likely it is to show up."

Sleep Suggestion: *Quiet the mind and calm the body by doing the 4-7-8 breathing technique. Simply, very slowly, inhale into the belly for a count of four. Hold your breath gently for a count of seven. And then exhale slowly, drawing your belly in, for a count of eight. The entire cycle takes nineteen seconds, putting your respiration rate at a very low and slow three cycles per minute. Your heart rate and blood pressure will decrease, getting you to your optimal sleeping heart rate, and your stress response will switch off.*

SLEEP TRAP #4: SLEEP-DISRUPTING HABITS

Each sleep stage is crucial for rejuvenating the body and brain. During Stages 1 and 2, muscles relax and start to be restored. During Stage 3, you produce human growth hormone, heal tissues, and undergo the glymphatic process of infusing the brain with nutrients and flushing out toxins. REM sleep is for consolidating memory and processing emotions.

A sleep cycle takes you on a journey through all these important stages. The body knows what it needs and allots sufficient time in each stage accordingly. We tend to frontload deep sleep earlier in the night and have longer REM periods during the last third. Short sleeping overall means you might wind up getting less REM. That would be a shame. You need a balance of all four stages for total rejuvenation. A short nap or just lying down for a few minutes can give you a dose of light and deep sleep healing. But you get REM only at the end of the cycle.

Short sleep steals REM time. But it's not the only culprit. Anything that deprives you of precious REM is to be avoided at all costs.

One REM thief is **alcohol** within two hours of bedtime. Now, it's true that having a glass of wine can be relaxing and might help you drift off to sleep. The problem is, alcohol makes you skim the surface of sleep. You wind up bouncing around in light sleep. In one waking hour, you can metabolize a cocktail or beer. It takes as much as four times as long to metabolize alcohol while sleeping.[21] That pre-bed wine could linger in your system until the second half of the night, keeping you in light sleep when you're supposed to be in REM.

A big meal within a few hours of bedtime is associated with overnight wake-ups, resetting the sleep cycle back to light stages, and depriving you of deep sleep and REM. The worst is **spicy food**. If you eat chicken vindaloo close to bedtime and lie down with a full stomach, heartburn is all but certain. It's hard for anyone to fall asleep with acid creeping up their throat. The resulting insomnia means less sleep overall, and less REM. Foods and beverages that contain **caffeine**—coffee, chocolate, soda, tea—close to bedtime take a wrecking ball to your sleep stages. Same problem here: Fewer hours of total sleep mean fewer hours of mental and emotional processing during dreamtime.

Do I even need to say that **cigarette smoking** is bad for sleep? It messes with hormonal rhythms. Nicotine is a stimulant that can cause insomnia. Smoking affects breathing, which can cause or exacerbate sleep-breathing disorders like OSA.[22]

Some recreational drugs might help you nod off, but that doesn't mean the sleep you get is the good stuff. Regarding **cannabis** (legal for recreational and medicinal use in thirty-eight states as I write this), CBD and THC products can definitely help you conk out and float you on a cloud into deep Delta-wave Stage 3 sleep. In one study, for 65 percent of users, CBD products immediately improved sleep.[23] However, high-dose cannabis products reduce REM time.[24] If you take a gummy before bed for a few weeks in a row and then stop, you might have some very strange and eerily vivid REM-rebound dreams.

With many **prescription medications**, you run the risk of suppressing REM. But those very same medications, such as **sedative-hypnotic drugs** like zolpidem (brand name Ambien), might help you get to sleep in the first place. **Beta blockers** for patients with a heart condition and alpha agonists for high blood pressure reduce REM, but they also keep you alive.[25] So . . . choices.

Sleep Suggestion: Physical pain is one of the most common causes of sleep deprivation. Fortunately, OTC nonsteroidal anti-inflammatory drugs (NSAIDs) such as Aleve and Advil and acetaminophen products such as Tylenol do not disrupt REM sleep. So if you have a headache or a backache, taking an occasional pill is fine. For extra help, you can try the PM varieties with antihistamines, which can make you feel drowsy. A capsule of Advil PM contains 38 mgs of diphenhydramine citrate, along with 200 mgs of ibuprofen. A tablet of regular-strength Tylenol PM contains 500 mgs of acetaminophen and 25 mgs of *diphenhydramine hydrochloride. Don't take any medication that makes you feel drowsy unless you are on the way to or already in bed. Long-term use (more than three times a week for more than two weeks) is NOT advised. There is now data directly linking the nightly use of diphenhydramine antihistamines and development of dementia later in life.*[26]

SLEEP TRAP #5: HOPING THE PROBLEM GOES AWAY ON ITS OWN

Sleep disorders are not made-up conditions that will magically disappear if you ignore them. By some estimates, as many as seventy million Americans have a sleep disorder, and I promise you that most do not seek professional help until their symptoms (some listed below) are alarmingly severe.

- Difficulty falling asleep
- Frequent wake-ups overnight
- Falling asleep at odd times
- Daytime fatigue
- Mood changes
- Difficulty concentrating or paying attention
- Frequent fatigue-caused accidents and mistakes
- Loud snoring or gasping for breath during sleep
- Muscle weakness
- Tingly or itchy sensations in the legs

Like many serious medical conditions, sleep issues can be diagnosed only with testing by a trained professional. Googling isn't going to cut it. If you suspect you might have a sleep disorder, bring it up with your primary care physician or family doctor. Best case scenario: You don't have one and can go about your life making minor tweaks to your routine to improve sleep quality and quantity. If you do get a diagnosis, that's good, too. You can go from there to treatment. You'll feel much better quickly when symptoms are reduced or eliminated. And you'll cut your risk of conditions associated with sleep issues, such as obesity, diabetes, stroke, heart disease, kidney disease, and depression.

There are eighty-eight distinct sleep disorders, according to the latest edition of the *International Classification of Sleep Disorders* (ICSD-3) manual. This book is hundreds of pages long. If you want to learn about all eighty-eight disorders, read it. I'm going to cover just the six most common categories, very briefly. If any of these sound like what you're experiencing, make a doctor's appointment today to find out for sure.

- **Insomnia** tops the list. It's the most common and widespread sleep problem and the number one reason that people seek the advice of a medical professional. Estimates are that 10 percent of adults have clinically diagnosable insomnia.[27] In short, insomnia is a catch-all term for, e.g., not being able to fall asleep at the beginning of the night, waking at 3:00 a.m. and struggling to go back to sleep, and waking at 5:00 a.m. and failing to drift off again before the alarm goes off. For some, insomnia is short-term and circumstantial, meaning that times are hard and you lie awake because of what you're going through. When things settle down and life goes back to normal, you can sleep untroubled again. For others, insomnia is a chronic condition based on your genetically determined chronorhythm. Dolphins deal with insomnia—to lesser and greater degrees—throughout their lives.

- **Sleep-related breathing disorders** affect between 2 and 4 percent of adults. The best-known disorder in this category is **obstructive sleep apnea (OSA)**, or paused or shallow breathing while sleeping due to an airway blockage. Some people with OSA stop breathing entirely for a few seconds, sputter awake gasping for air, and then go back to sleep—multiple times per night...and they might not even know they're doing it. **Central sleep apnea** is a cessation of breathing due to a brain signaling problem, not an obstruction. **Hypoventilation** sleepers breathe too slowly and shallowly to get enough oxygen and wind up with carbon dioxide overload.

- **Circadian rhythm sleep-wake disorders** are not necessarily related to chronotypes. They're more commonly linked with age and behaviors. For example, seniors can dose off right after dinner and wake up before dawn. Adolescents can sleep until 2:00 p.m. on Saturdays when you want them to get up and clean their rooms. Overnight shift workers whose bodies refuse to sync up with their schedule—about one third of America's fifteen million shift workers—might suffer from **shift-work sleep disorder**. Symptoms include poor-quality and -quantity sleep, headaches, extreme fatigue, impaired executive functioning, body aches, mood swings. You might be familiar with these symptoms if you travel internationally. **Jet lag disorder** occurs when your body is in one time zone but your circadian rhythm is in another.

- **Hypersomnolence** means being overtired and relates to several disorders suffered by the chronically exhausted. **Narcolepsy**, for example, a hypersomnolence disorder that affects 1 in 2,000 people, makes people drift off uncontrollably, at random times. (FYI: Chronic fatigue syndrome can look like hypersomnolence, but is actually not a sleep disorder. Excessive tiredness is a symptom of this multisystem illness.)

- **Parasomnia** is when you walk, eat, have sex, and drive while falling asleep or actually asleep. **Sleepwalking** is the best-known parasomnia, and highly likely to be a plot twist in a murder mystery. It's possible to get out of bed, walk around, have full-blown conversations, clean a closet, or drive to the supermarket, shop, and put the groceries away, while asleep. When the sleepwalker wakes up, they might have no memory of what they did, including have sex.
- **Sleep-related movement disorders** include twitching and moving your limbs, grinding your teeth, or clenching your jaw while you're asleep. **Restless legs syndrome**, when you have an intense impulse to move your legs despite trying to rest and fall asleep, might be accompanied by itchy sensations. **Nocturnal leg cramps** cause sudden, painful spasms in the feet or calves as you're lying in bed, ready for sleep.

To get a diagnosis for any of the above, go to your doctor. They will start by asking you a series of questions about your symptoms, list of medications, underlying conditions. Answer honestly. Sleep is a litmus test. If you are healthy, you sleep well. If you don't sleep well, it could be a sign of trouble. I can't tell you how many times the info in a standard sleep questionnaire led me to connect the dots and discover another issue that needed to be treated immediately, and that treatment saved the patient's life.

If you've been keeping a sleep diary, take it with you to your doctor's appointment. There may be diagnostic clues in there, too. Get a blood test to check for any deficiencies (I like to look at vitamin D, magnesium, iron, and sometimes melatonin). A doc might recommend an at-home sleep apnea test. Depending on severity, you might need an overnight sleep study, called polysomnography, in a lab. Nothing to be nervous about. It's noninvasive, painless, and very useful.

Once you have an official diagnosis, you and your doctor can design a treatment plan for your specific issue. Medications or supplements like melatonin or magnesium for sleep-onset problems might be recommended. Cognitive behavioral therapy for insomnia is highly effective and helps Dolphins get the most sleep they can reasonably hope for.

For breathing disorders, surgery might be necessary for obstructions. But most likely, you will be prescribed a continuous positive airway pressure (CPAP) machine with a little mask that goes over your nose and pumps pressurized air into your airway to keep it open while you sleep or an oral appliance—a specialized mouth guard—that will slightly move your lower jaw forward, opening up your throat.

Circadian rhythm disorders such as jet lag can be eased with bright light therapy that tricks your master clock in the hypothalamus into thinking it's on a different schedule. Go to timeshifter.com for guidance about how to minimize symptoms and get back in sync.

For teeth grinding and jaw clenching, you might have to get used to wearing a mouth guard at night. I have one patient, a Dolphin, who is very sensitive to light and sound, so he wears an eye mask and earplugs to sleep. When I diagnosed him with teeth grinding, he had to wear a mouthpiece, too, and mouth tape to keep it from falling out. His wife started calling him Tommy.*

---

*   Millennials and Gen Zers: *Tommy* is a movie. Look it up or ask your parents.

SLEEP DOCTOR FINDER

How do you even find a sleep specialist in your area?

Most people have never even considered seeing a sleep specialist, but if you want to, here are a few ideas to get you started:

- Talk with your GP or primary care doctor, who may refer you to a good sleep specialist.
- Call your insurance provider to ask about specialists and requirements for doing a sleep study. Insurance policies often cover in-network sleep studies.
- Ask someone you know who has a sleep disorder.
- Go to sleepcenters.org.

Apart from treatment for sleep disorders, what can you do to quickly improve the quality and quantity of sleep, to get that domino down, and the others that follow?

You know what to do. Keep reading.

TAKEAWAYS

- The consequence of not enough, and not good enough, sleep is steep. Whole-body balance is all but impossible without it.
- Illness. Inflammation. Insatiable tunger (tiredness + hunger). Irritability and tanger (tiredness + anger). It's all likely on insufficient sleep.
- Not to mention anxiety, depression, and emotional regulation issues.
- Knowing your chronotype—Bear, Lion, Wolf, or Dolphin—can change your life and sleep habits for the better. Go to chronoquiz.com to learn yours.

- Once you know your chronotype, you can calculate ideal wake times and bedtimes and get in sync with your genetically determined rhythms.

- Top sleep disrupters: inconsistent sleep schedules (including sleeping in on weekends), alcohol, caffeine, nicotine, pre-bedtime screen exposure, pre-bedtime snacking, drinking water right before bed (and having to get up to pee in the middle of the night).

- You might have a sleep disorder without realizing it. Don't pretend fragmented sleep, chronic insomnia lasting longer than three months, or waking up exhausted are normal. If you have doubts, talk to your doctor—not Dr. Google!—about your symptoms. If needed, discuss treatment options.

CHAPTER 4

Sleep for the Win

Snooze your way to glorious good health by sticking with five simple rules. Remember, wellness is simple, if you focus on fundamentals! Get the sleep domino down and you will reap whole-body rewards.

SLEEP DOMINO GOODIES

stronger immunity
reduced inflammation
more energy (and a hot bod)
weight loss
mental sharpness
longer life
more fun in bed

TOP FIVE TIPS FOR BETTER SLEEP

Be consistent.
Shift some things.
Set the scene.
Nap for the win.
Accept awakeness.

A well-rested person lives in a completely different body compared to someone who doesn't get enough, or good enough, sleep on a constant basis.

A huge internal benefit to being a good sleeper is **stronger immunity**. The production of white blood cells and anti-inflammatory cytokines peaks during overnight sleep hours.[1] A good sleeper's immunity army is always on the march, weapons drawn and ready to fight germs and free radicals. While you're horizontal, defender cells amass in lymph nodes — 600 to 800 nodules located all over the body, which filter bacteria and other hazardous materials — knocking out pathogens before they can make you sick. Antibodies — protein antidotes that neutralize specific viruses and germs — are formed mostly during sleep hours. What's more, according to a 2020 study, being a good sleeper boosts the effectiveness of antibodies in vaccines,[2] giving you an extra coat of armor.

Sleep Science: The body is well aware that sleep increases your defenses against harmful invaders. So when a virus takes hold and your immunity army mobilizes to do battle, it sounds an alarm that signals to the brain that you need to go lie down. During sleep, the immunity army is fortified and can move more quickly into battle position. That's why, when you get sick, you feel so damn sleepy. So listen to your body when it tells you, "Go lie down!"

Reduced inflammation. Immunity and inflammation go together. When you have an injury or an infection, white blood cells rush to the site to fight back. That rush of blood swells up the area, inflaming it. That's healthy and normal. The trouble comes when inflammation doesn't recede. The "all clear" signal gets jammed, leading to chronic inflammation. According to a 2022 study, reducing participants' sleep by ninety minutes per night for six weeks changed their DNA defender cells. There were too many of them, and they were less effective. A larger, bumbling immunity army increases inflammation and makes things worse. Good sleep prevents overproduction, so the right number of immunity cells go to the right place, kill invaders, and leave. Infections are destroyed without gumming up the works.[3]

More energy. Good sleepers are more likely to exercise.[4] The relationship between exercise and sleep is bidirectional, meaning both behaviors beget the other. So if you are a non-exerciser who struggles to fall asleep, adding a few weekly workouts or vigorous walks might be the missing piece of the puzzle to get you to the magical 450 minutes of nod per night.

Some people are just not interested in exercise, I get it. There have been times in my life when fitness wasn't a priority. But if you are looking for a solution to the problem of low-quality sleep, exercise might be the right prescription for you. When you start getting adequate sleep, you will have more energy and *want* to go to the gym. You won't have to make bargains or bribe yourself to do it or contend with guilt when you don't.

If you are new to regular exercise, get the domino of sleep down first, and you'll be shocked at how fast you find time and motivation to move. Sleep also helps you tone up faster. During deep Stage 3 sleep, burgeoning muscles get a chance to recover from that day's workout, making you stronger and ready to go again. You really can sleep yourself stronger.

> **Sleep Science**: Good sleep helps you maintain muscle mass, even while you attempt to lose fat. For a University of Chicago study, researchers divided their overweight

middle-aged nonsmoking participants into groups: one that had an 8.5-hour opportunity for sleep, and the other that had only 5.5 hours of sleep time. For the next fourteen days, both groups stuck to the same diet. The group that slept 8+ hours per night enjoyed more energy and decreased appetite. They lost 55 percent more fat and retained 60 percent more muscle mass compared to the low-sleep group.[5]

Weight loss. Sleep is like free Ozempic. It curbs appetite. If one of your health goals is to drop a few pounds, stop counting carbs and count sheep instead. Sufficient sleep increases leptin (the satiety hormone) and decreases ghrelin (the hunger hormone). If you are well rested, you're *far less likely* to reach for empty-calorie, carb-heavy snacks and drinks for quick energy.

TIRED + HUNGRY = TUNGRY

But when tungry (tired and hungry), your defenses are down and your hormones are out of whack. So you wind up eating processed foods, which then trigger intense cravings for *more* processed foods.[6] Being well rested eradicates tunger, and the pounds fall away.

Smarts. You can nurture your genetic baseline intelligence with education and brain-stimulating activities like puzzles. But even if you never play Connections, you can stoke your gray cells and blaze new neural pathways just by sleeping well. If you thought staying up all night studying before a big test was a smart strategy, you were wrong. During sleep, your brain consolidates memory. It puts everything you learned that day into filing cabinets in your subconscious in a logical order so that when you need to retrieve that information, your brain knows where to find it. Learning itself—problem solving and processing information — is enhanced by REM when electric signals are zipping along your brain's eighty-five billion neurons and their synapses.

Arts. Synapses are like bridges, connecting neurons and allowing them to talk to each other. By sleeping, you gain new understanding and get all your brilliant ideas. What is creativity, if not the brain coming up with novel concepts? REM is the key to unlocking creativity.[7]

> ***Sleep-Creativity Hack***: *In 2023, researchers at MIT had some of their participants wear a device that tracked their sleep stages while taking a forty-five-minute nap. At sleep onset, they were prompted to dream about a tree. After having a dream, they recorded a description of it. A control group stayed awake for the same amount of time and were told just to think about trees. Once the forty-five minutes ended, both groups were asked to do a few tasks, including a storytelling task: writing a tale that used the word tree. The dreamers came up with far more creative stories than the awake subjects. They also scored higher on "divergent thinking tasks," such as listing things you can do with a tree and making quick noun-verb associations. Researchers found that, across the board, "tree"-prompted dreamers were 78 percent more creative than their awake counterparts.[8]*

Longer life. To prove the sleep-longevity connection, in 2023, an international team of researchers collected data from nearly 61,000 male and female participants from the United Kingdom, average age sixty-two, to calculate a Sleep Regularity Index. After adjusting for lifestyle and other health factors, the researchers found that subjects with higher sleep regularity were found to have a 20 to 48 percent lower risk of death from all causes, a 16 to 38 percent lower risk for cancer death, and a 22 to 57 percent lower risk for heart-related death. They also found that, to predict mortality risk, sleep regularity was more important than sleep duration.[9] (Remember what I said about resetting your circadian rhythms on the weekend? Yeah.)

Hot Sleep-Sex Suggestion: *To have more fun in bed, sleep on it. These two behaviors have a lot in common. Like sleep disorders, sexual dysfunction is rife in America. As of 2020 data, 33 percent of men and 45 percent of women have some degree of dysfunction.[10] Sex and sleep each have four thrilling stages. You know the sleep stages by now. Sex stages are desire, arousal, climax, and resolution. Sleep and sex have a bidirectional relationship. When one behavior is good, the other is likely to be as well. Regarding desire and arousal, longer sleep duration – even just one hour more – translates into next-day desire and greater genital arousal in women.[11] Poor sleep quality correlates with lower sexual satisfaction.[12] Sleep disorders such as insomnia and OSA can lead to sexual problems such as erectile dysfunction.[13] Perhaps the most important sleep-sex nexus is intimacy. If partners are sleep-deprived, they get tangry (tired + angry), and the ensuing conflict does not put them in the mood for love.[14]*

To enjoy all these benefits, you must fix sleep first. It's not hard. If you try these Top Five Sleep Tips, you will get that domino down.

SLEEP TIP #1: BE CONSISTENT

The science shows that consistent sleep-wake patterns whittle your waist, prolong life, and promote sleep. If that's not enough for you, setting wake-up times and bedtimes just makes your life simpler and eradicates one source of stress: anxiety about getting enough sleep. When you stick with a schedule, even on the weekends, you train your brain to fall asleep faster, stay down all night, and wake up during REM or light sleep, sparing you the brain fog and uncomfortable punch-drunkenness of sleep inertia (that's feeling like a truck hit you when your alarm wakes you out of deep sleep).

Establish a consistent wake time. Stick with it every day, including Saturday and Sunday. After two weeks, you won't need to set an alarm. If you have flexibility with your work and social schedule, **choose a wake time that's in sync with your chronorhythm.**

Quick reminder:

Bears' "jump-start" hormones—cortisol, insulin, and testosterone—start flowing two hours before natural wake time, gently tapping the gas, signaling the body that it's time to start the day. **Bears' natural wake time is usually 7:00 to 7:30 a.m.**

Lions' hormonal shifts begin two hours earlier and are more pronounced. **Lions' natural wake time is usually between 5:00 and 6:00 a.m.** It might be dark out, but Lions are ready to *go*. No snooze button needed.

Wolves' hormonal shifts start later, making their **natural wake time between 8:00 and 9:00 a.m.** They might have to rise earlier for work or social reasons, putting them at risk for waking during non-REM sleep, with resulting sleep inertia. Wolves are just not designed to function before 10:00 a.m. or until the brain fog clears. They can move that along by increasing heart rate and cortisol release with a burst of upon-waking exercise and direct sunlight.

Dolphins have upside-down hormonal cycles. Their cortisol is *lower* in the morning than it is at bedtime and overnight.[15] Dolphins' circadian rhythms conflict with social and professional norms. Given their challenges, my recommendation is that **Dolphins wake up between 6:00 and 7:00 a.m.**

> *Strong Sleep Suggestion*: One more time, I want to be clear about this: If you do only one thing for your overall sleep quality than anything else, wake up (based on your chronotype) each day at the same time!

Establish a consistent bedtime. After a week or two of establishing a set wake time, get in sync with your chronorhythm for bedtime as well. For the big three chronotypes, bedtime is calculated as eight hours before wake time, which gives them a half-hour to drift off and still get 7.5 hours of sleep.

Bear bedtime: 11:00 to 11:30 p.m.

Lion bedtime: 9:00 to 10:00 p.m.

Wolf bedtime: midnight to 1:00 a.m.

Dolphins, again, are a special case. Because their blood pressure, body temperature, and cortisol don't drop at nighttime, they don't feel sleepy at the appropriate time to get in bed. Since a good night for them is six hours of rest, I recommend that they get in bed around **11:30 to midnight** to limit overall in-bed time, thereby preventing some staring-at-the-ceiling anxiety and frustration.

EASY BEDTIME CALCULATOR

To calculate the perfect bedtime for your schedule, regardless of your chronotype, start with the time you have to wake up, and count backward. So if you must rise at 7:30 a.m., get in bed by 11:30 p.m. to give yourself thirty minutes to fall asleep and net 450 minutes of sleep. If you know that it takes you longer than thirty minutes to fall asleep, make bedtime thirty minutes sooner and try again for a week.

One last complication to factor in is the number of minutes of wakefulness throughout the night. It's completely normal to wake briefly between cycles. If you are older and have had alcohol or more than five ounces of any beverage within three hours of bedtime, you might make a trip to the bathroom in the wee (as it were) hours.

Do your cats jump on your head at 3:00 a.m. every night, waking you up? Does your dog hog the bed? Add up every minute of overnight wakefulness and subtract that sum from your bedtime. So if you need to get up at 7:30 a.m. and generally experience fifteen minutes of overnight wakefulness, your updated bedtime would be 11:15 p.m., fifteen minutes earlier.

SLEEP TIP #2: SHIFT SOME THINGS

As an ice cream addict, I'm the last person on Earth to tell people to cut back on anything that gives them joy. But to get the sleep you need, you might have to rearrange the timing of your consumption of sleep-interfering substances and activities.

Caffeine intake. The timing of coffee continues to fascinate TV hosts and podcasters. Every time I do a media appearance, I get asked about this.

**For all chronotypes,
I recommend coffee with lunch
instead of breakfast.**

The reason coffee makes you feel less tired is that it helps to clear the drowsiness chemical adenosine from brain receptors. When you first wake up, though, those receptors have already been cleared by sleep. Regardless of what you might believe, all morning caffeine does for you is make you jittery.

Here's the science: In order to wake up, your body has to produce two hormones—adrenaline and cortisol. When it does that, your brain becomes highly stimulated. If you compare coffee to adrenal hormones, it's like weak tea to cocaine. All caffeine will do to you is give you some side effects. But if you wait ninety minutes after you open your eyes to have your first cup, you will get more bang for your buck.

If you shift caffeine to lunchtime, it blocks adenosine and temporary stalls your sleep drive for a few hours to get through the rest of the afternoon. No coffee, tea, or caffeinated soda after 3:00 p.m., though! Give your body plenty of time to metabolize the caffeine out of your system completely by bedtime.

Dinner time. As previously mentioned, eating spicy food too close to bedtime can cause sleep-disruptive acid reflux. Drinking alcohol with that spicy meal interferes with REM. If you are used to eating late—sitting down to eat dinner at 9:00 p.m. in the European tradition—consider changing your schedule to eat earlier. Ideally, each chronotype would take their last bite of the day (and sip of alcohol) four hours before their set bedtime.

Bears should finish eating by 7:00 p.m.
Lions should finish by 5:00 or 6:00 p.m.
Wolves and Dolphins should put down the fork by 8:00 p.m.
If you stick with this dinner schedule, you will reinforce your chronorhythm for hunger, digestion, *and* sleep.[16] It might be a

challenge not to snack after dinner when you eat early, but only at first. After three or four days, your system will adjust and cravings will diminish.

Water intake. Your kidneys have a chronorhythm, too. They are most active from morning until afternoon. But around dinnertime, the brain starts secreting antidiuretic hormone, which makes the kidneys slow down, filter less blood, and produce less urine.[17] The system was designed this way so you don't have to get up and urinate every few hours overnight. But just because the kidneys slow down when it gets dark does not mean they stop functioning. If you drink a lot of water, they will produce urine, day and night. This becomes a problem if you get up to pee two or more times per night consistently. Fragmented sleep is low in quality. The simple solution is to shift water intake. Be mindful about hitting your daily hydration goals before dinnertime. If you do have a beverage after dinner, limit it to five ounces, and sip slowly. Last, know that alcohol inhibits the brain from releasing antidiuretic hormone. So wine, beer, and other booze block the hormone that slows kidney function. Put another way, you may pee like a racehorse, regardless of the time of night, when you drink alcohol.

Exercise. If you leave work at 6:00 p.m., have a quick bite to eat, then head to the gym at 8:00 and run on the treadmill until 9:00, you are working (out) against your best interests. Vigorous exercise within three hours of bedtime elevates cortisol and adrenaline, heart rate, core temperature, blood pressure — all the markers that need to *decrease* for sleep. And if you do manage to fall asleep despite a heightened core arousal marker, your sleep efficiency — spending adequate time in all four stages, especially REM — could be compromised. NB: Wolves are the exception to this rule. According to a 2023 international study, evening-preferring athletes who exercised at high intensity at 7:30 p.m. retained "stable" sleep efficiency despite the timing of their workouts.[18] Morning- and intermediate-preferring athletes? They took a sleep stability hit.

Shift workouts to earlier in the day. At night, if you need to do something, try light yoga or stretching that quiets the sympathetic nervous system and produces the feel-good hormone serotonin. When serotonin goes up, cortisol goes down, creating the perfect balance before bed.

Screen time. When our ancestors lived in caves, the only light that pinged their optic nerves after dark came from the moon, stars, and fire. Cycles of sunlight and darkness kept the brain's master clock in sync. When night fell, our ancestors' endocrine and cardiovascular systems downshifted into physiological processes that culminated in sleep.

Modern humans don't have it so lucky. When darkness falls for us, artificial lights go on in every room, confusing the master clock into thinking it's still daytime. As you must have heard, the blue light from phones, watches, TVs, and computer screens suppresses melatonin production. Those in cities have no escape from streetlights and bright signage. Even if you live on top of a mountain, your circadian rhythm could be affected by artificial light when you open the refrigerator door or check the glow of a digital clock.

It'd be ridiculous to advise anyone to limit all artificial light and screen time within three hours of bedtime, when melatonin should start its nightly drip. Those hours are, for many, their only opportunity to catch up on personal emails, watch TV shows, and explore social media. If it's not possible to shift those activities, do what you can to take in less light. Move the couch farther away from the TV. Use a blue-light blocking filter on your devices. And commit to turning off the screens at least an hour before bed.

Sleep Suggestion: Everyone needs a runway to land the plane. I ask all my clients to establish a Power-Down Hour. This adds a little structure to your evening, which will get you to bed on time relaxed and with the best chance of *getting quality sleep. Make a habit of taking an hour before bed to wind down. Consider it an electronic curfew to avoid all blue-light-emitting devices that block melatonin release. I chop up my Power-Down Hour into three segments. The first twenty minutes are for practical tasks, like tidying up or doing some paperwork. During the middle twenty minutes, I take a shower, floss, and brush my teeth. The last twenty minutes are for relaxation, journaling, and some light stretches.*

***Super-Secret Sleep Hack**: If you remove makeup at night or have a multistep skincare routine, take care of this earlier in the evening, because if you wait until just before bed, you will probably wind up in the bathroom with bright lights on, telling your brain it's morning rather than evening.*

SLEEP TIP #3: SET THE SCENE

Your bedroom is not *just* a bedroom. It's an environment that can either help or hinder sleep. The five words you need to remember to set the stage for sleep: dark, cozy, quiet, cool, and humid.

Dark. As dark as you can make it. You don't have to buy blackout curtains. But you can secure your curtains with a hairclip or chip clip. Make sure ambient light doesn't come in under the bedroom door. Invest in a decent eye mask that fits comfortably and snugly. Don't worry about every blue or red light on small electronic devices, just the bigger offenders.

Cozy (and Clean). There is no way to objectively measure coziness level. You know it when you feel it. Does snuggling up in bed make you go, "Ahhhh"? Your sleep space should fill you with a sense of security and peace. The bed itself should be enticing, with clean sheets and plumped pillows. For this reason alone, I urge everyone to make their bed each morning so that it's inviting at night. Of course, comfort is key. Mattress firmness and pillow profile are individual choices that only you can make for yourself. If you are in the market for a bed or pillow, swing over to sleep doctor.com, where we have done a lot of the hard work for you, with over 150 reviews and tests. A between-the-knee pillow helps with back alignment and adds a layer of comfort. Warning: If you associate your bedroom with anything besides sleep and sex, it might not have such cozy associations. So never do anything stressful (like work) in the bedroom! If you get into an argument with your partner in there, stop immediately and take the fight into a different room.

Quiet. Noise tolerance for sleep varies from person to person. But it's rare for anyone to drift off in a loud room. If you are particularly sensitive to sound, try earplugs or a white noise machine. The key is "continuous noise," a consistent hum, per a 2020 study.[19] Sleep-disrupting noise is a sudden change, like the blast of a car horn, an alarm clock going off—or a sudden eerie quiet.

Cool. The optimal temperature for sleep is 65 to 70 degrees Fahrenheit.[20] If you have a thermostat in your bedroom, set it accordingly. As needed, turn on the AC in the summer and open your window a crack in the spring.

Humid. Air quality affects sleep because if the room is too dry, it can irritate your throat and nose and interfere with breathing and relaxation. Thick, wet air isn't ideal for breathing, either. Allergens, mold, and pollutants hang in the air and get sucked into your lungs, causing nighttime coughing and congestion. Plus, excessive humidity can make you sweat. Soaked sheets and PJs are not cozy. According to the Environmental Protection Agency, the ideal indoor humidity level is 30 to 50 percent.[21] Some thermostats have a humidity function. You can estimate indoor levels by looking at outdoor levels on a weather app. If your bedroom is too dry, use a humidifier, and get some plants! Green friends need misting, and naturally make any space more jungle-like. If bedroom air is too thick, turn on the AC or a dehumidifier. Consider an air filter for your bedroom. You are breathing that air for six to eight hours a night; it's better if it's clean.

> **Sleep Sense**: *Bedroom rehab suggestions address four of the primary senses:*
> *Sight: Decrease light.*
> *Hearing: Eliminate noise.*
> *Touch: Set temperature and get cozy.*
> *Smell: Have clean and humid air.*

SLEEP TIP #4: NAP FOR THE WIN

I am a big fan of napping, especially when watching golf on TV. Napping is a delicious way to pay down some sleep debt. I want to be absolutely clear that taking a nap can't undo the negative effects of chronic sleep deprivation or provide the same restorative power of a full night's sleep. Assuming that you can make up for bad sleep with a nap is like saying a light afternoon snack provides the same nutritional value as a balanced dinner. Also, remember, if you have difficulty falling or staying asleep, a nap will reduce your sleep drive and may make insomnia worse. I tell my insomniac patients to never nap!

Different types of naps can help achieve different goals. An "essential nap" helps you recover from an illness or an injury. A "fulfillment nap" allows babies and toddlers to hit their sleep goals during the developmental years. "Recovery naps" help curb fatigue after a bad night. A "proactive nap," aka "disco nap," is a planned rest earlier in the day to bank sleep so you can dance the night away like Barbie and Ken without unattractively yawning.

Length matters when it comes to napping. Short naps lasting fifteen to thirty minutes can increase alertness, boost immunity, and lower stress.[22] According to a 2021 study, a ninety-minute nap improves cognitive performance, especially if you are chronically sleep-deprived.[23] But daily naps for older adults, especially those longer than ninety minutes, are associated with increased risk of medical conditions like hypertension,[24] diabetes,[25] and cognitive impairment.[26]

The best time to nap is in the early afternoon, siesta time, between 1:00 and 3:00 p.m., when most chronotypes have a natural cortisol drop called the "postprandial dip." A quick snooze during that window clears the accumulated adenosine in your brain to give you a second wind of energy and alertness to get you through the rest of the day without disrupting your nighttime sleep. Just remember, it can be harder to wake up from a longer nap. Make sure to give yourself extra time to fully awaken before getting back to important work tasks. If you nap too long or wake up in the middle of deep sleep, you'll wake up groggy with sleep inertia, as if you're still half asleep. That feeling can take hours to shake off.

Some nap rules to rest by:

Choose the right environment. A quiet, dark, private space is perfect.

Schedule your naps. Just like set bed-wake consistency, scheduling a nap at the same time each day will make it easier to drift off quickly and wake up when you want to.

Set an alarm! Otherwise, a catnap might turn into a hibernation.

Nap Hack: I call this trick a Nap-a-Latte. Right before your nap, drink a cup of coffee (a small beverage will have about 100 mg of caffeine, the amount you want for this). The

> *caffeine will kick in twenty or thirty minutes later, right when you've planned to wake up, and help erase any trace of grogginess. You'll be restored, clear-headed, and ready to go for about four hours.*

Wolves and Dolphins know all too well that taking an afternoon nap might feel good in the moment, but they will pay a heavy price for that at bedtime, when their usual struggles to doze off at an appropriate hour are worse than usual. They need to build up sleep pressure all day long to conk out at night. Any release of that pressure with a nap will keep them up and lead to fatigue the next day — and a greater temptation for a siesta. You can see how vicious sleepless cycles might get triggered by a seemingly harmless little nap.

The best time to nap is approximately seven hours after waking. The optimal nap timing for each chronotype:

Bears. Since you wake at 7:00 a.m., **the ideal nap time is 2:00 p.m.**

Lions. Since you wake at 5:00 to 6:00 a.m., **the best nap time is noon to 1:00 p.m.**

Wolves. Since you wake at 8:00 to 9:00 a.m., **you could nap at 3:00 or 4:00 p.m.**, but I wouldn't recommend it. Sorry, furry friends. Your schedule skews later already, and if you nap that late in the afternoon, it could delay sleep onset, setting up a night of deprivation.

Dolphins. Do not nap! Your goal is to improve the duration and quality of sleep *at night*. Taking an afternoon nap is self-sabotage. If your energy levels drop midday, take a walk or jump up and down to get your heart rate, blood pressure, and cortisol level elevated. Or go outside and expose your optic nerve to sunlight, which signals the brain, "Yup, still daytime!" In fact, whenever you lose steam, train your brain to think, "Exercise and sunlight."

SLEEP TIP #5: ACCEPT AWAKENESS

Every previous tool in the sleep box has been about discipline and strategy.

The last tool for getting the sleep domino down is a bit different. It's making a mental and emotional shift that might be difficult for type A people (like Dolphins and Lions) who expect results if they do what they're supposed to do.

> *Sleep Science*: In 2024, Australian researchers published a study in Sleep about insomnia during a particularly stressful time, namely, the COVID-19 pandemic. More than two thousand participants reported on several factors over a twelve-month period. Insomnia trends emerged in the data. The subjects with persistent insomnia had high levels of "sleep reactivity" and "sleep effort," which means they were stressed out about how hard it was to get to sleep. The more stressed out they were, the less likely it was for insomnia symptoms to go away.[27]

When you are doing everything right, and sleep still goes wrong, practice acceptance. There will be instances when the strategies just don't work.

> *My Sleep Story*: If I'm lying in bed, super anxious about a personal or work thing, there's no universe where I'm going to fall asleep. If I just accept that reality, it'll lower my anxiety about not sleeping, and in doing so, I just might drift off after all. Or not. I often tell myself, "You've had sleepless nights before, and you will again. And you're fine."

Even as we aspire to improve our wellness and get dominos down, we have to cut ourselves some slack. There will be times when you do sleep in on the weekends, and that's okay. I have no doubt that, on occasion, you will eat and drink wine very close to bedtime. You will overnap, stay up late, scroll social media in bed, and commit every sleep sin in this (and any) book. And I'm here to tell you, it's okay. Dolphins and Lions with sleep issues really beat themselves up about not doing everything right. And I tell them, "I personally don't sleep perfectly; in fact, there are times when I don't sleep well, and I'm the Sleep Doctor. Everyone just needs to give themselves some slack."

Accept that bad sleep happens on occasion. Forgive yourself if you have self-sabotaged. The beauty of it is that you always get another chance to get it right the next night.

Right about now you may be wondering, Is that it? What about the program to assess my sleep and fix it? Don't worry, it will all come together, but before I lay it all out, we have two other Dominos to discuss, starting with Drink.

TAKEAWAYS

- When you sleep better, you feel better. You *are* better!
- With sleep-boosted immunity and reduced inflammation, you're less likely to get sick.
- With improved mental function and emotional regulation, your professional and social lives will seem easier and more satisfying.
- Set wake times and bedtimes based on your chronotype as best you can, given the demands of daily life, to get in sync with your natural biology.
- Adjust the timing of exercise, dinner, and alcohol consumption (avoid for three hours before bed, in most

cases) to improve the chances of drifting off without effort.

- Your bedroom is your sleep sanctuary. Make sure it's dark, cozy, quiet, cool, and humid.
- Napping can help you pay off some sleep debt, if you plan naps strategically based on your chronorhythm. Keep naps short and sweet.
- Sometimes bad sleep just happens. Accepting this truth alone takes the pressure off and makes it easier to go back to sleep or sleep well the next night.

DOMINO TWO

drink

Simplify health and wellness by getting
the second fundamental biobehavior down.

CHAPTER 5

Drink 411

You need to continually replenish your body with fluids for all your organs and systems to function. In this chapter, soak up buckets of knowledge about hydration, aka Water Wisdom!

WHY IS HYDRATION SO IMPORTANT?

HOW DOES THE BODY KNOW IT'S HYDRATED?

WHY DOES DEHYDRATION HAPPEN?

HOW DOES QUENCHING WORK?

HOW LONG CAN YOU SURVIVE WITHOUT DRINKING?

After sleep, hydration forms the second most important domino of total body wellness. In pursuing your wellness goals, you're more than welcome to drink all the green juices, shell out hundreds of dollars for a new workout set, or throw away your entire snack drawer to start clean on Monday; *or* you could start simple with an easy daily water-drinking routine to kickstart some healthy habit forming and get you on track to making decisions that are geared toward your long-term health. We all want to feel better in our bodies and in our skin: This second domino will have you feeling both, and in spades.

So let's dive right in.

I want you to picture a kitchen sponge.

When it gets wet, the sponge absorbs water. Even when you wring it out, some moisture stays in it for a while. In the morning, when you go to the kitchen to make your breakfast, you plainly see that, overnight, due to evaporation, the sponge has dried out completely. It's also smaller because it has lost the fluid that added volume. In the absence of that fluid, it shrinks. A completely dry sponge is pretty much useless. If you tried to clean a dish with it, you'd wind up smearing the grease around and making a bigger mess than you started with. To rehydrate the sponge and make it useful again, just add water. At first, the dry sponge will resist absorbing the water, and a lot of it will run off. But with enough fluid, the sponge holds the water until it's saturated. When it can't hold any more water, the water just runs off again.

Your body is a flesh-and-blood kitchen sponge. When it's hydrated—replenished with water—it's plump and functional. When it's dehydrated—deprived of water—it's dried out, shriveled, and useless. Add inadequate water, your body is only semi-functional. Too much water, and your body will just eliminate the excess.

Human hydration is that simple, while also being very complicated. The biology of hydration, and the mechanisms inside the human body to keep our flesh-and-blood sponges moist, is one of the most fascinating systems we've got, as you'll soon see.

WHY IS HYDRATION SO IMPORTANT?

We need water because we are water. The human body is 60 percent water. Along with blood and lymph—80 and 96 percent water, respectively—your muscles are mostly water, too, at 76 percent. Seventy-five percent of your brain and heart are made of water. One of the driest parts of the body, your skeleton, is 22 percent water. Cartilage is at 80 percent. Even fat is 10 to 30 percent water.

If there were no water-filled cartilage cushions between your bones, they would grind against each other, causing terrific pain.

Without adequate fluid in the spaces between skin cells, you wouldn't be able to sweat, and would overheat to the point of fainting.

Water maintains blood volume so it can flow with enough force through your cardiovascular system to deliver glucose, protein, and oxygen to cells. Dehydrated, thick blood trickles sluggishly through vessels, depriving your organs and tissues of nutrients. It's called a blood*stream*, not a blood*ooze*, for a reason; we need it to flow smoothly.

The heart is more water than muscle; it pumps blood that every cell in the body needs for replenishment and repair. If you're dehydrated, your heart shrinks and is less powerful, and struggles epically to pump thickened blood.

The digestive system uses water to break down food into proteins, fats, carbohydrates, and vitamin and mineral molecules, which are absorbed by the spongey small intestine and transported into the bloodstream. The colon walls need to stay moist with viscous mucus so that stool can glide through the intestines on its way out of the body. Otherwise, stools get stuck. The number one cause of constipation is dehydration.

Water provides a medium for the metabolic process, which your cells are engaged in 24/7. All those chemical changes—like converting sugar into energy—don't happen in a vacuum or on dry land; they happen in water.

Cerebrospinal fluid floods your central nervous system (the brain and spinal cord) with nutrients so that it can regulate every life-sustaining function in the body. This fluid, as part of the glymphatic system, also sweeps the brain of toxins and cellular waste every night.

If the lymphatic system becomes stagnant from dehydration, the detoxifcation process is affected, and cellular waste piles up inside the body, leading to inflammation and illness.

Without adequate fluid intake, your body struggles to perform *all* these essential functions we need to live—and many more.

HOW DOES THE BODY KNOW IT'S HYDRATED?

The human body has a system that constantly monitors the ratio of fluid to electrolytes (sodium, potassium, magnesium, calcium, chloride, among others) in the bloodstream and makes constant adjustments to keep the ratio balanced. This system is called "water regulation homeostasis" or "osmoregulation." *Osmosis* refers to the movement of water through a cell membrane. Osmoregulation controls the movement of fluid throughout the body. The major organs involved in this process are the brain and the kidneys, with a big assist from key hormones.

The brain's hypothalamus is the master gland that controls circadian rhythms, hunger, mood, body temperature, heart rate, everything that needs to stay in balance to function well—including hydration.

The hypothalamus knows when you're dehydrated because (1) it shrinks (in fact, the entire brain shrinks when even moderately low on fluids), and (2) the concentration of electrolytes, primarily sodium, in the blood is too high. In response, the master gland signals the nearby pituitary gland to secrete vasopressin, aka antidiuretic hormone. This hormone sends an all-systems alert to conserve fluid and tell the kidneys to slow down and to use less salt (and draw less water from tissues) in its blood filtration process.[1] The kidneys continue to filter blood and produce urine. But since they're using less water to do it, urine becomes more concentrated and changes from pale yellow to a darker shade of yellow, even orange.

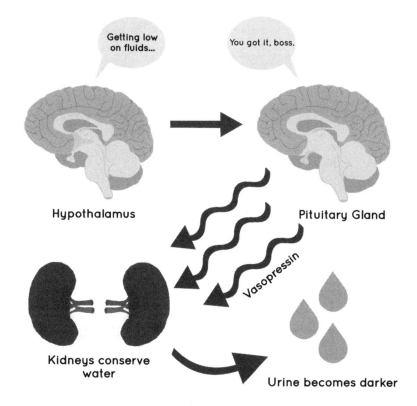

The dehydration alert begins in the brain, moves to the kidneys via the endocrine system, and, within seconds, your body conserves fluid to reset the water-sodium ratio and get back into homeostasis. You might notice a change in urine color, but otherwise, you'd have little idea all this is going on. Meanwhile, your thirst command center — the hypothalamus-pituitary complex — is always monitoring and tweaking fluid levels.

The osmoregulation system also works in reverse. If you have too much water in the body, blood volume increases. That leads to a rise in blood pressure and a shift in the water-salt ratio in the opposite direction. The hypothalamus notices overhydration because (1) the brain swells, and (2) sodium concentration is too low. In this case, the master gland will signal the pituitary to *suppress* vasopressin. The kidneys get the message and use more salt in the blood filtration process, pulling the extra fluid from surrounding tissues and producing diluted urine. As a result, your pee will be pale yellow or clear and you'll be running to the bathroom more frequently than usual.

WHY DOES DEHYDRATION HAPPEN?

Hydration means replenishment. And dehydration means inadequate replenishment. If you are dehydrated, you are not doing a good job of replacing the two or three liters of water you lose every day through sweat, breath, urine, and feces. When you cut yourself, you lose water through blood. Even the act of blinking, which we do around 15,000 times per day, causes water loss. It's not a lot, but every drop counts.

Conventional wisdom says that if you are a healthy adult with access to clean water, you are unlikely to become dehydrated. However, water loss can happen to health-conscious people due to circumstances beyond their control:

- Having an impaired thirst mechanism (and not knowing it)
- Having mental health issues that make you ignore physiological signals
- Conditioning oneself to ignore physiological cues
- Living in a tropical or desert climate
- Working outside in the heat and not taking (or being allowed) water breaks
- Sweating profusely from exercise and forgetting to replace fluids and electrolytes
- Taking diuretics or laxatives
- Having a condition such as kidney disease or Addison's disease
- Having an acute GI condition that causes excessive vomiting and/or diarrhea
- Taking thirst-suppressing medications for hypertension or depression

Granted, severe dehydration in healthy adults with access to water is unlikely. Inadequate hydration, on the other hand, is common. Per 2017 data, in the U.S., as many as 29 percent of adults are underhydrated, with Black, Hispanic, and low-income people at highest risk.[2] Between 17 and 28 percent of older adults are likely to experience clinical dehydration.[3] In the over-seventy bracket, 95 percent of men and 83 percent of women aren't drinking enough.

Mild dehydration or underhydration might not kill you. But its symptoms will interfere with your life, happiness, and health. If you have been having headaches, brain fog, a lousy mood, fatigue, weakness, and muscle cramps for no apparent reason, it is probably because you aren't drinking enough water.

HOW DOES QUENCHING WORK?

After a long walk on a hot day, it's so satisfying to gulp down a big glass of water. The water hits the back of your throat, and you feel instantly quenched.

But how can that be? The water hasn't even reached the stomach yet, much less the intestines, where it is absorbed into the bloodstream to pump up volume and eventually reaches the brain with a water-salt ratio update. That process—lips to brain via the guts—takes ten to fifteen minutes. So why is it that we feel rehydrated before thirst is, in fact, quenched, and why do we stop drinking—usually after one minute—before the brain registers the replenishment?

At the California Institute of Technology, a research team studied quenching dynamics to get answers to those very questions and published their findings in 2019.[4] They looked closely at nerves that line the mouth and throat. When a person is dehydrated, the brain signals to those nerves to start twitching, giving you a "must drink now" feeling called a "gulping signal."

If you are thirsty, your brain is telling you to drink. As soon as liquid washes over those nerves, they send a signal to the brain to turn off the thirsty feeling and to dole out a hit of feel-good hormone dopamine, like a thank-you note for hydrating. That dopamine is so satisfying that the gulping signal is cut off after about one minute. You put down the glass, wipe your mouth, and say, "Ahhh. I needed that." Otherwise, you would continue to chug for the entire ten to fifteen minutes it would take for blood volume to increase and the brain to register that you are, indeed, rehydrated. The researchers concluded that the one-minute stopgap "satiety signal" is nature's way of preventing animals from drinking too much in general or too much of a nonhydrating liquid.

From your mouth, fluid travels down the esophagus, into the stomach, and through the small intestine and the colon. When it reaches the guts, nerves in the digestive tract assess the water concentration in the beverage you just drank and send a report upstream to the brain. If the beverage was insufficiently hydrating, the brain reactivates the gulping signal, making you thirsty again.[5] You might think you can fool the thirst command center by doing shots of tequila. But you would be wrong. The gut-check hydration mechanism makes sure that you keep drinking until you're replenished.

> ***Water Wisdom****: The dominant thirst cue is physiological. But some thirst cues are behavioral, like going to a cocktail party. The first thing the host asks you after you walk through the door is, "What can I get you to drink?" Anticipating this social custom, it's likely you felt thirsty the whole way there.[6] It's the same thing when you sit down at a restaurant and the server fills a glass with water. I don't know about you, but I reach for it instantly and take a gulp whether I'm thirsty or not. For hydration's sake, use social conventions of hydration to your advantage, and never refuse a hydrating beverage.*

HOW LONG CAN YOU SURVIVE WITHOUT DRINKING?

Although the body can cling to fat cells for decades, it can't hold on to water for a single day. You can die after just three days without water. "Hydrate or die-drate" isn't just a cheeky phrase people say to each other at the gym. It's the truth.

The three-days rule is not cut-and-dried (out). There was a case in 1979 of an Austrian man named Andreas Mihavecz surviving for *eighteen days* without food and with barely any water. What happened to this poor bastard is the stuff of a horror movie. Mihavecz was eighteen, a bricklayer's apprentice who was a passenger in a car crash. Three local cops locked him up in a holding cell in the local jail, presumably in order to get his statement about the crash. Each of the three cops assumed that one of the others had let Mihavecz out of the cell, but none had. He was locked up in that basement cell for two and a half weeks, despite his mother's pleas for answers, until another officer noticed a putrid odor coming from the basement. When Mihavecz was discovered, he was in a sorry state. He'd lost over fifty pounds and had to be hospitalized for weeks. The bumbling cops who'd accidentally left him to die were fined (whatever the amount, it wasn't enough). Mihavecz got a settlement from the city, and his story became legend. The guy endured a nightmare that few of us can imagine suriviving. The key to his survival was that he'd licked condensation off the grimy walls of his prison.

If you're curious about what happens to the body when it's depleted of water, here's a day-by-day breakdown:

After one full day without water, a person will lose 2 percent of their body weight in water and feel increasingly thirsty. The gulping signal will start clanging, making the throat painfully parched. Without incoming fluid, the body clings to what it's got already. All outgoing water processing — sweating, peeing, crying, pooping — slows down. Since sweat cools the body, your body temperature may go up. Whatever urine comes out will be disturbingly dark. Blood volume decreases, making it harder for red blood cells to deliver oxygen and nutrients to hungry cells. Under strain, your heart pumps harder and breathing rate increases.

After two days without water, you'd be down 4 percent in body weight. What does a drop like that look like? If you weigh 150 pounds, you'd be down six pounds. It might not seem like much, but that water weight makes a huge difference to your circulatory system. To keep the bloodstream moving, water is sucked out of surrounding tissues and cells and redirected into blood vessels, providing nutrients to the brain and heart to maintain vital functions. But even so, blood pressure drops, causing dizziness and fainting. Skin feels uncomfortably dry. Lips crack. Since you've stopped sweating, in warm conditions you get hotter and hotter without the ability to sweat and cool down.

After three days without water, you'd be down 7 percent of your body weight in water and start to look like a kitchen sponge in the morning. Dried out and shriveled. Because of extreme electrolyte imbalance, you are at risk for seizures and cardiac events. The gut stops functioning. The body's filtration systems—the kidneys, liver, and lymphatic system—grind to a halt, causing sludgy cellular waste and toxins to pile up throughout the body. The dehydrated organs and tissues that sent water into the bloodstream to preserve life dry out and start to die themselves, resulting in organ failure. Your brain is the last to go, which is truly the stuff of nightmares.

I'm not a hydration alarmist, per se. But even mild dehydration can have consequences. The best way to be sure you stay hydrated is to know if you are down a pint or three. Good thing there are easy, free ways to check your hydration level in the very next chapter.

TAKEAWAYS

- Hydration means replenishment with water, the substance that makes up most of your body. Without replacing water that's lost from sweating, peeing, crying, etc., your organs and cells can't do their jobs.

- It's all about maintaining the essential ratio of water to sodium and other electrolytes. Your brain's thirst command center does the regulating for you, but you can help yourself by responding to signals that tell you, "Drink now!" by having a big glass of water.

- It's true that you'd die after three days without drinking at all. And it's not a pretty death. Your body will shut down, system by system, organ by organ, until you are a shriveled husk.

- Even slight dehydration—down 2 percent of your body weight in water—can negatively affect your health and knock you out of whole-body balance.

CHAPTER 6

Drink Assessment Tools

Before you can knock down the second
Domino of Wellness, check your hydration
status with these at-home tests.

URINE COLOR TEST

THE PINCH TEST

SELF-REPORTED THIRST DISCOMFORT RATING

Hydration testing is sort of like glucose testing. A simple lancet test with a meter and test-strip reveals a snapshot of blood sugar in that very moment. A more sophisticated A1C test from a blood sample provides in-depth data on blood sugar over the last two to three months.

The at-home tests in this chapter reveal snapshot information about your hydration level. But to test for chronic or severe dehydration, you need to go to the doctor and get a battery of tests, including heart rate, blood pressure, and blood volume, and give samples of blood, urine, saliva, and tears. More invasive tests are called "neutron activation analysis" and "stable isotope dilution," which are super accurate but pricey and, honestly, not necessary for 99.99 percent of people. If you are determined to get the most revealing and scientifically calculated assessment of your hydration, by all means, check your plasma sodium level. Look into the ratio of nitrogen and creatinine in your urine. Have at it!

Or . . . you can just go to the bathroom.

URINE COLOR TEST

The most noninvasive technique ever: Look at the hue of your urine in the toilet bowl. Google "Indonesia hydration color chart" to see a color guide created by researchers in Indonesia, which has a tropical climate where staying hydrated is a serious concern. Clear or pale yellow means you are hydrated. Golden hues are fair. When you move into orange and brick, it means you are dehydrated.

The issue with using urine color as a fail-safe assessment tool is that it doesn't necessarily show how close to homeostasis your system is. The more concentrated your urine, the darker the color. The more diluted it is, the lighter the color. Pale yellow or nearly clear urine does show that it is diluted, usually indicating a healthy hydration level. However, it could also mean that your kidneys are dumping urine to rebalance the all-important water-salt ratio. Gentle reminder that hydration doesn't *only* mean adequate fluid intake. It's all about the homeostatic balance of internal fluids and electrolytes. You can't tell from urine color alone that you are in balance.

BEYOND THE PALE

Urine should be clear, pale yellow, buttery yellow, or golden. When you move into the amber, sunburst, and tangerine hues, have a tall glass of water ASAP.

But what if your urine is a shade other than yellow or orange? Pee of another color is most likely caused by medications or by brightly colored foods or beverages. But in some cases, vivid urine might be a neon warning sign that you need medical attention.

- **Neon yellow**. You are probably taking too much supplemental vitamin B12 (riboflavin). Cut back on that for a day or two and see if your urine returns to normal.
- **Neon orange**. A likely culprit is eating a boatload of vitamin A–rich foods such as mangos or carrots. Or it could be due to the urinary tract infection (UTI) medication phenazopyridine or the tuberculosis medication rifampin.
- **Dark orange**. First, rule out dehydration by drinking 16 ounces of room-temperature water. If your urine is still dark orange three hours later, you might be overdoing it with magnesium supplements. Otherwise, if you are drinking plenty of water, dark orange urine could indicate liver disease such as acute viral hepatitis or cirrhosis.
- **Red**. Have you had beets, rhubarb, or blackberries recently? If so, that's probably the cause. Of course, red could mean blood, and that is never good. You might

have a UTI, kidney stone, or urinary tract cancer. Taking senna for irritable bowel syndrome or constipation can also turn urine a muddy red. If you take senna, go off it for a few days.

- **Green**. Asparagus can turn pee slightly green. The arthritis medication indomethacin and the anesthetic drug propofol can, too. If you have a severe UTI populated by a certain type of bacteria, your urine may be lime colored.

- **Bluish green**. Blame medications again. Cimetidine treats ulcers and acid reflux and can turn urine teal, as does the antidepressant amitriptyline and the pain reliever indomethacin.

- **Blue**. Blue urine is almost certainly caused by food coloring. Or you've been to the hospital and had your kidneys or bladder tested by drinking dyes. Blue pee is NOT a sign that you're losing your mind, as the sovereign in *The Madness of King George* does. Historians believe George III's urine turned (royal) blue because he was being treated with a gentian, a plant with intensely blue or violet flowers.

THE PINCH TEST

I'm a dog and cat lover and have spent a lot of time in veterinarians' exam rooms checking on the health and wellness of my pets. Small dogs in particular are at high risk for gastrointestinal issues that cause severe dehydration. A vet can tell in two seconds if a dog has fluid loss by pinching the fur on the back of its neck. If the scruff snaps back into place right away, the dog is not dehydrated. But if it takes more than a few seconds, the pup needs a subcutaneous injection or intravenous fluid ASAP. Another quick vet test is to touch a dog's gums with the tip of a finger. If the finger sticks—like a tongue on a cold flagpole—the dog is dehydrated.

The gum test isn't accurate for people. And, last time I checked, humans do not have a furry scruff to pinch. But we do have skin, and strategical pinches in certain places can test "skin turgor," or elasticity, that does indicate whether you are hydrated at any given moment. A few caveats with this method: It works best on younger people. Skin becomes less elastic as we age, so the over-sixty crowd's skin will stay in the "tent" position longer than a twenty-year-old's. And because of variables—how long should you pinch before release? Exactly how fast should the tent snap back?—the skin turgor test isn't considered by scientists to be the most accurate assessment tool.

However, on a hot day or after a sweaty gym session, if you want a quick check of how hydrated your skin is, try this:

1. Lightly pinch the skin on the back of your hand for three seconds.
2. Let it go.
3. Count how many seconds it takes the skin to return to normal. Less than two seconds indicates you are hydrated.[1] Longer than that, you could have water loss that needs to be addressed.
4. Repeat fifteen minutes after rehydration.

SELF-REPORTED THIRST DISCOMFORT RATING

In 2023, scientists in Erzincan, Turkey, published data on a "Thirst Discomfort Scale"[2] that helps caregivers make an accurate assessment of the hydration needs of patients at risk for dehydration due to their conditions and medications.

In a nonclinical setting, like at home, you can self-assess by asking some of the same questions on the scale. Thirst is the body's way of telling you that you are mildly dehydrated. Since busy, harried people (as in, "I don't have time to hydrate!") have conditioned themselves to ignore thirst cues, learning to self-assess thirst is a new health practice you didn't think you needed, but sure do. It takes two minutes to mentally run through the questions and can be repeated throughout the day. (NB: Assessing thirst discomfort isn't a reliable tool for people with dementia or those recovering from brain injury or stroke.)

On a scale of 1 (not at all) to 4 (intensely, yes), rate the following statements:

1. My mouth and throat are dry.
2. My lips are dry.
3. My saliva is thick.
4. I have a bad taste in my mouth.
5. I want water.

SELF-REPORTED THIRST DISCOMFORT SCORING

Add up the numbers you gave (1 to 4) for the five questions above.

5 to 9: **Hydrated**. You are probably not suffering from dehydration. But check again later and keep sipping fluids.

10 to 14: **Mildly dehydrated**. You should take a break from whatever you're doing soon, however important and engrossing it might be, and drink a glass of water.

15+: **Dehydrated**. Stop what you're doing and sip 16 ounces of water right now. Drink another 8 ounces every hour until dinnertime. Get in the habit of drinking more every day from now on so you don't become dehydrated again.

WHAT ABOUT FREQUENCY AND VOLUME?

The color of urine is a great indicator of hydration. But the frequency and volume of urination isn't necessarily.

For one thing, "normal" **urinary frequency** depends on so many factors — age, race, gender, location, etc. — that it's very hard to say what a normal range would be for you, without a discussion or meeting. There is some data about general metrics. For a 2022 large-scale study[3] of nearly 2,000 healthy women in the Boston area, researchers asked participants to track their daytime and nighttime urination frequency. Some interesting findings:

For healthy women:

Number of daytime bathroom trips: two to ten

Number of overnight bathroom trips: zero to four

For "elite healthy" women with strict dietary and fitness routines:

Number of daytime trips: two to nine

Number of overnight trips: zero to two

Older women (45 to 64) peed more than younger women (31 to 44).

Black women tend to pee less often during the day and more often at night, compared to white women.

Those who drank more water peed more during the day (no surprise there), but overnight, the quantity of fluid intake didn't really matter. The well-hydrated peed just as often as the underhydrated. (This has to do with the kidneys slowing down at night per their circadian rhythm.)

But it's not only hydration that can cause you to pee a lot. For people with certain medical conditions, frequency goes off the "normal" charts.

- **Diabetics'** kidneys can be overwhelmed by the job of processing high glucose levels in the blood and so dump excess sugar into urine. As a result, they pee often and at great volume, in a condition called polyuria.
- An **overactive thyroid** brings on a slew of symptoms, from insomnia to brain fog to out-of-control hunger — and increased urination.
- **Kidney stones** are a less common (600,000 cases a year in the U.S.) condition that increases frequency, with a side order of severe pain and bloody urine. I don't think I need to urge anyone to see their doctor if they have kidney stones; if you have one, you are probably running (and crying) to the ER. The pain is horrific, radiating down the back and throughout the pelvis. You may pass kidney stones on your own, painfully, or they can be treated with outpatient surgery.
- **Pregnancy**, especially in the third trimester, causes increased frequency because of hormonal shifts and the fetus doing the rumba on the mother's bladder. Excessive peeing may continue postpartum, due to the body naturally releasing fluid retained during pregnancy. If you are still peeing more than ten times a day a month postpartum, tell your doctor.
- Men with **an enlarged prostate**, aka benign prostatic hyperplasia (BPH), feel the need to urinate frequently because the oversized walnut-shaped organ puts pressure on the bladder. They might have to urinate every hour or two, especially at night.

- The most common cause of frequent urges is a **urinary tract infection**. According to the Urology Care Foundation, UTIs account for eight million doctor visits a year and are the second most common bodily infection. Although men do get UTIs, they are far more common in women, due to the shorter length of the female urethra (the pee hole) and its closer proximity to the anus. Most UTIs are caused by bacteria migrating from the anus to the urinary tract. How to tell if you have one: Do you feel an intense urge to pee but release only small amounts and experience a burning sensation? Ding, ding, ding. Consult a physician *immediately* for treatment. You can prevent UTIs by wiping front to back, drinking plenty of water, and urinating after intercourse. But the only way to cure one is with prescription antibiotics.

- **Seniors** naturally produce less antidiuretic hormone than they did when they were younger, so their kidneys receive a weak signal from the master gland to inhibit urination overnight. So the older you get, the more you have to get up and pee during the night.

On the "frequent urination does not indicate hydration" theme, it needs to be said that frequent peeing does not indicate *dehydration*, either. Some beverages just make you pee a lot, which isn't a bad thing... or a good thing either.

- **Alcohol**. Say you went all day without drinking much water at all, and then, at the bar that night, you downed two pints of IPA quickly. Soon, you will feel the urge to go to the restroom. After "breaking the seal," you might need to relieve yourself every fifteen minutes thereafter.

Beer does seem to pass right through a person. And it does seem to make you pee as copiously as the mountain stream on the bottle's label. Alcoholic beverages suppress antidiuretic hormone. As a result, the kidneys produce beer-bucket-loads of urine, uninhibited. But don't worry: You won't pee out much more than you put in.[4] Alcohol is close to a net-zero beverage, neither hydrating nor dehydrating. If you are a rosé-all-day person, worry about your liver. But your water-salt ratio will be okay. Since you do lose a little fluid from alcohol, have a glass of water between units of wine or spirits.

- **Coffee.** A hot mug of joe is a net-zero beverage, too.[5] I was surprised by the research on this because I'd heard my whole life that caffeine is a diuretic. It is, but you have to take in a lot of it. Drinking 180 mgs of caffeine — around two eight-ounce cups — will not affect your water-salt ratio. Go ahead and count two coffees or caffeinated teas toward your daily hydration goals.[6] They will make you pee more ... but only because you consumed fluid. Now, if you go up to three cups per day, you will have crossed into potentially dehydrating levels of caffeine.

- **Soda.** Caffeinated or decaffeinated, soda does not make you urinate more liquid than you consume. It's still liquid sugar in a fizzy form. The calories and glucose spike are not worth the hydration. If you love carbonation, drink unflavored seltzer.

So alcohol, coffee, and soda are not as terrible as you thought, hydration-wise. But a net-zero beverage is still not as good for you as a zero-calorie, zero-sugar, net-hydrating one, like seltzer, water, or herbal tea. I would never tell anyone to completely stop drinking beverages other than water. Just as your body is always reaching for homeostasis, you have to strike a balance, too. But I recommend that you limit non-water beverages to one or two per day.

As for **urinary volume**—how much you pee—that does provide information, but not really accurate data on hydration per se.

> **Water Wisdom**: *For any mammal over 6.6 pounds, urine streaming duration – how long it takes to empty the bladder – maxes out at twenty-one seconds.[7] In 2014, a Georgia Institute of Technology mechanical engineer named David Hu published his study about animals in the Atlanta zoo. Regardless of size, urethra width, bladder capacity, or urine stream pressure, the animals, from elephants to horses to cats, all peed for roughly the same length of time. I call this the 21-second rule.*

Now that you know about the 21-second rule, I dare you not to count seconds as you pee. It feels like a small triumph to get to nineteen or twenty seconds, smug in the knowledge that the bladder is reaching its full potential.

There are some exceptions to the 21-second rule. Men with benign prostatic hyperplasia (BPH) might not have much of a urine stream to speak of. The enlarged prostate squeezes the urethra, which narrows the passage and partially blocks or slows the flow of urine out of the body. They might feel that full bladder but can't evacuate it for twenty-one continuous seconds. Instead, they'll likely do it in short spurts.

If you pee for less than twenty-one seconds, it means you're voiding a less than full bladder. An urgent need to pee that results in a small yield could be the sign of a UTI. Go to your doctor to confirm or rule it out.

If you pee for *longer* than twenty-one seconds, it probably means that you lack opportunities to void when the bladder is full—a common phenomenon among teachers and nurses—which can result in a stretched bladder. If you feel that your bladder is full, empty it. You don't win any prizes for holding it in. If anything, you might win yourself a UTI.

What matters is normal urinary frequency and volume *for you.* If you notice a sudden increase in how often and how much you pee, it probably means you are hydrating more... if it's not a symptom of diabetes. If you find yourself peeing less, it probably means you aren't drinking as much as usual... or you have an enlarged prostate.

Any sudden changes should be reported to your doctor. The Dominos of Wellness are litmus tests for general health. Part of the Big Picture lesson of this book is to pay closer attention to things you take for granted to bring your overall health and wellness into focus. And that includes what you see when you look inside the toilet bowl.

TAKEAWAYS

- Checking your hydration level is easy and free. No doctor's office visit required.
- Look in the toilet after you pee, and if you see any color other than clear or pale yellow, go have a glass of water. Rainbow pee color is most likely due to food or medication, but it could indicate illness, so if you pee red and haven't had beets, call your doctor.
- The pinch test: not just Instagram folklore. Pinching the skin on the back of your hand to check for snap-back speed is a useful, quick hydration test. If the skin takes

longer than two seconds to return to a normal position, have a drink.

- Peeing a lot doesn't necessarily prove you're hydrated or dehydrated. But constant urination could mean you have diabetes. The constant urge to go could mean a UTI or an enlarged prostate. Get those symptoms checked by a doctor.
- Turns out coffee (up to two cups) and alcohol are not dehydrating. They're "net-zero" liquids, meaning you pee out about the same amount as you put in. Plain water is more hydrating. Try alternating net-zero beverages with water, e.g., one coffee, one water; one cocktail, one water.

CHAPTER 7

Troubleshooting Drink

Fill a glass with water, raise to lips, and drink. Hydration doesn't have to be all that complicated. And yet, most of us have some kind of drinking problem.

THE CONSEQUENCES

low energy
poor physical performance
poor mental performance
headaches
low blood pressure
constipation
joint pain
increased disease risk
dry skin

THE TOP SIX DRINKING PROBLEMS

forgetting to drink
choosing not to drink
drinking too much
not sleeping enough
mistaking bloat for hydration
drinking unfiltered tap water

I've seen a few examples of people suffering from severe dehydration right in front of me, and it was kind of shocking. I'm not a big yoga person, but I tried CorePower Yoga with my daughter in a small class wall-to-wall with people in a hot room, and everyone was doing all kinds of yoga moves. You leave drenched in sweat, looking as if you fell into a swimming pool. Students take sips from their water bottles throughout the practice, but if you start in an underhydrated state, sipping during class won't be enough to replenish lost fluids.

When the class ended, the instructor opened the studio door, letting cool air rush in, which felt wonderful. I rolled up my mat and went to hang out in the lounge area to drink some water and recover from the workout. As I sat on a cushioned bench, I watched another student, a 30-year-old woman, stagger out of the hot room, apparently disoriented. She reached for the wall for support, but her hand slid across it. She lost her balance and fell to the ground.

I jumped up to help and rushed over along with a few other people. She hadn't just slipped. She was flat-out unconscious on the floor. Although she came to after just a few seconds, she was shaken. The instructor and I insisted that she sit on a bench and sip a bottle of electrolyte-infused water slowly over the next half-hour. When her dizziness faded, she laughed about it. "I do this class three times a week and always drink a liter of water beforehand. But today, I was rushing to get here from work, and didn't have time to drink. I thought I'd be okay." The lesson for her, and for me, was that you can't mind-over-matter your water-salt ratio.

Another time, I was walking through a southwestern American city on a very hot August day with a small group that included a seventy-five-year-old man. Our guide had urged us to bring water bottles on the two-hour sightseeing tour. I happened to notice that the elderly gentleman wasn't sipping from his bottle like everyone else, and I asked him about it. He said, "I've never really liked to drink water. I'm fine without it. People say I'm part camel." Well, by the second hour of the tour, this man's face had turned bright red, and I thought he might be having a cardiac event. He asked to take a break from walking and sat down on a park bench. When the rest of the group was ready to move on, the man said, "I can't get up." His legs were cramping, and his hands were trembling. The tour guide did not hesitate. He immediately called for an ambulance. When it arrived, the EMTs started an IV saline drip to rehydrate him. Later that day, the guide sent an email to the entire group, assuring us that the man was fine. He was "just" dehydrated. I guess he wasn't part camel after all.

As I said, I am not an alarmist about hydration like many experts (and influencers) who say that you need to drink a gallon of water a day to stay hydrated. But I'm not on the side of experts who say things like "If you get hungry, eat. If you feel thirsty, drink. Your body knows when you need to hydrate." Hydration *is* intuitive, absolutely. But the two stories above show you that staying hydrated often needs to be an intentional act. Because of modern life, we can't rely on the powerful third command center in the brain to maintain fluid level. Another part of one's brain—the know-it-all part, the so-busy-with-other-things part—might think it knows better and that you can get away with not drinking. Hydration isn't always convenient. But you can wind up paying a high price for not prioritizing it.

A quick rundown of the consequences of underhydration (a chronic state of being down a pint or two) and dehydration (an acute state of being down at least 2 percent of your body weight in water) and how they can sabotage your day, life, and health.

Low energy. Inadequate fluid makes you drag, not only because your cells are slow to receive energizing nutrients due to lower blood volume. Dehydration is associated with fatigue[1] because when you're low on fluid, sleep is shorter and lower in quality.

Poor physical performance. Athletes who are hydrated with fluid and electrolytes run faster and jump higher than their dehydrated counterparts, in study after study.[2] It's not even subtle. For one 2018 analysis, researchers intentionally dehydrated athletes with heat intervention until they had lost 3.2 percent of their body weight in water. After a three-hour recovery period when they were allowed to eat and drink, the athletes were asked to perform demanding exercises. Compared to the control group, the dried-out group just couldn't keep up. Their strength and endurance were severely affected, and they felt exhausted.[3]

Poor mental performance. Even water loss of just 2 percent in weight affects concentration, memory, executive function, and energy level in men[4] and women.[5] If you didn't drink for a day and a half before a big test, how do you think you'd do? A 2019 Chinese study explored this very question. After thirty-six hours with no water (but plenty of food), the subjects were given math tests. They didn't do well. On top of a high error rate and poor concentration, they had "low vigor" (everything felt like a slog) and "low affect" (a bad mood). After they had rehydrated, they took another test an hour later and showed improvement across the board.[6]

More headaches, including migraines.[7] Brain shrinkage hurts. When your brain gets smaller due to water loss, nerves all over the organ are compressed. (Overhydration can also give you a headache for the opposite reason. The brain swells inside the skull, causing painful pressure.)

Low blood pressure and dizziness. Ever feel woozy when you stand up? One possibility is dehydration.[8]

Trouble in the bathroom. Constipation is a major symptom of dehydration. If you are dehydrated, the colon sucks water out of stool to hydrate itself. As a result, feces become hard nuggets that don't slip-and-slide through the already dry colon.[9] Chronic dehydration can bring about other elimination miseries, such as kidney stones and UTIs.

Joint pain and inflammation. When you are dehydrated, the body takes fluid away from nonessential parts and moves it into the bloodstream to keep you alive. Much of that water is taken from connective tissue, including the synovial fluid that lubricates joints. By draining the cushioning, your joints go from looking like fluffy pillows to empty pillowcases. The ensuing friction as bone grinds against bone causes inflammation and pain.

Increased disease risk. In reports on scientific studies, you hear a lot about "associations." Dehydration might not directly cause disease the way cigarette smoking causes lung cancer, but you can find a lot of research about conditions, such as diabetes, heart disease, kidney disease, and Alzheimer's disease, that are associated with poor hydration.

Dry skin. It doesn't seem like much of a consequence compared to terrible diseases, but it sure can be annoying, even painful.

> **Water Wisdom**: *Just a 2 percent drop of your body weight due to dehydration from a workout or not drinking enough leads to the loss of flexibility of your blood vessels, a precursor to atherosclerosis, aka hardening of the arteries. In a University of Arkansas–led international study, researchers tested the effects of dehydration and found significantly impaired blood vessel function.[10] The participants in the study were not grizzled old folks with craggy arteries, but ten healthy men in their mid-twenties with springy vessels.*

So what bad habits are responsible for chronic underhydration and acute dehydration? According to my research, the Top Six Drinking Problems are as follows:

DRINKING PROBLEM #1:
FORGETTING TO DRINK

I get it. Life comes at you really fast, and it's all too common for people who are just fighting to keep their heads above water to forget to stop and sip. In a distracted and harried mental state, you might not notice cues from the thirst command center that say, "Drink now!" You're focused on a work deadline, or getting to school pick-up, or fixing the leak in the sink. Over time, you become habituated to ignoring biological cues. Before long, you're not just ignoring them; you don't even notice them.

Dehydration due to busy-ness is a complex problem. Even swamped people remember to have coffee upon waking and a glass of wine in the evening. The difference is, for many people, morning coffee and nighttime pinot are habitual behaviors with rewards built into them. The coffee rewards are the aroma, the flavor, the ritual, the jolt, the moment of peace and pleasure in an otherwise crazy day. The wine reward is all of that, minus the caffeine, plus a buzz. Objectively, water offers the best reward of all: It's quenching. It's hydrating. It is exactly what your body requires to achieve homeostasis. But in terms of flavor? It doesn't hold water, as it were.

Habits are automatic choices, things you repeat so often that you don't have to think about doing them. Habits do not spring fully formed into your life. They are made—and unmade—through repetitive behavior. For example, if you smoke one cigarette, you don't have a smoking habit. But if you smoked a pack a day for a few months, you'd make one.

Right now, if you don't have a water-drinking habit, only intention and repetition will create one. If you're already busy and stressed, the idea of adding another item to your "I really should..." list might have you reaching for another glass of wine.

DRINKING PROBLEM #2:
CHOOSING NOT TO DRINK

Some people choose not to drink because they just don't like doing it (shout out, Mr. "I'm part camel"). If you're on a long car ride, many people think it's a smart idea to limit beverage intake so you don't have to waste time by stopping to pee every hour or two. Some people don't drink water on airplanes to avoid awkwardly climbing over their seatmates and standing in line for the cramped bathroom. Women with bladder incontinence might choose not to drink so much before going to a funny movie if they know that laughing causes accidents.

Planned dehydration might seem wise. But in the long run, you'll do yourself more harm than good. Delaying trips to the bathroom on a long car ride can cause UTIs and stretch the bladder. The bladder is not made of rubber, though. Stretch it often enough and it will fail to contract and release urine as it should.

> ***Water Wisdom***: *Not drinking on airplanes is a great way to compound the effects of killer jet lag. I recommend 8 ounces of water for every hour in the air.*

Incontinent women who fear leaking at a comedy film must weigh the benefits and risks. The benefit is obvious. The risks of mild dehydration include brain shrinkage and cognitive impairment. You'll stay dry, but you might not get the movie's jokes. As an alternative, use incontinence products that prevent embarrassing situations.

Failure to replenish fluids can easily turn into a UTI. Among those 60+, especially women, a simple UTI can bring on serious symptoms. Quick story: A close friend's mother, age ninety, liked to sit on her deck in the sun and read all day. She refused to drink anything but coffee and gin. Her caregiver tried to get her to drink water, but she said, "At my age, I don't have to do anything I don't want to do!" Fair enough. But then the older woman started having strange symptoms. Her appetite, like her taste for water, was nonexistent. She was always tired. She had dizzy spells. It all came to a head when the caregiver drove to the store one mile away for groceries, leaving the older woman on the deck by herself. On the drive back from the store, the caregiver was shocked to see the woman walking erratically on the road. It was just good luck she wasn't hit by a car. The caregiver immediately pulled over and asked the older woman where she was going. She replied with a nonsensical word salad. Alarmed, the caregiver got her into the car and drove straight to the emergency room. The diagnosis was dehydration and a raging UTI that caused dementia-like symptoms. She had to be hospitalized overnight with a saline drip and antibiotics. The entire episode could have been avoided if the older woman had accepted the fact that hydrating is important.

DRINKING PROBLEM #3:
DRINKING TOO MUCH

Can you really drink too much water? Ask Brooke Shields.

According to a 2023 article in *Glamour* magazine,[11] Shields had been drinking excessive amounts of water to stay hydrated while preparing for a one-woman show in New York City. She was waiting for an Uber when she started to feel disoriented. She wandered into a nearby restaurant, and then, as she said, "My hands drop to my side and I go headfirst into the wall . . . frothing at the mouth, totally blue, trying to swallow my tongue." She blacked out in a grand-mal seizure. The story has a happy ending, though. When she came to in an ambulance, she had an oxygen mask on her face and the actor Bradley Cooper was sitting next to her. He'd been walking by the restaurant when she passed out and stayed by her side until help arrived. The seizure was caused by hyponatremia, an extremely low salt concentration in her blood, because she'd been drinking too much water. Once her water-salt ratio was rebalanced, she was fine. Shields told *Glamour* that her doctor's prescription was to "eat potato chips every day."

Water toxicity is exactly what it sounds like: being poisoned by too much water. Don't freak out. It's not going to happen to you if you chug a bottle of water or a can of beer on a hot day. You'll just pee or sweat out the excess. But if you consume a large quantity of fluid really fast and if you don't get rid of it via urination or perspiration, the kidneys just can't handle the volume of incoming fluid or get rid of the flood fast enough. The crucial balance between water and salt is thrown way off. The normal range for blood sodium is 135 to 146 millimoles (mmol) per liter. Go below 135 mmol, you're at risk of confusion and nausea. Drop a bit more, and you could have muscle spasms or a seizure, like Shields. When sodium levels drop below 125 mmol, a fatal brain edema is assured.

Every year, one or two water toxicity death stories make the news. I've heard about fraternity hazing incidents where pledges were forced to consume ridiculous quantities of water or unsafe social media "challenges" that have followers guzzle a vast amount of water in under a minute. Hydration challenges might seem like all fun and games . . . until someone winds up with brain swelling.

Again, this is not going to happen unless you down *a lot* of water very fast or consume a gallon or more every single day for days on end. I don't want to scare anyone away from hydrating adequately.

Those at highest risk for water toxicity: people whose kidneys are already compromised due to disease and extreme athletes who sweat out a lot of their sodium and then chug large amounts of water to replenish. Hyponatremia can be avoided by sipping electrolyte-enhanced water before, during, and after an intense workout.

Sleep Science Meets Water Wisdom: According to a 2019 international study, 20,000 adult participants in the U.S. and China who routinely slept for six hours a night were between 16 and 59 percent more likely to wake up dehydrated than their counterparts who regularly slept for eight hours a night. The proof was in the urine samples: Poor sleepers had more concentrated pee in the morning.[12]

DRINKING PROBLEM #4: NOT SLEEPING ENOUGH

Bad sleep and dehydration are a toxic combination.

You might think those who slept fewer hours would lose *less* water from overnight exhalation of vapor. Perhaps they do. But the association between short sleep and dehydration goes deeper than that, all the way into the endocrine system.

Vasopressin, a hormone, is secreted and suppressed throughout the day as the body continually monitors and adjusts the water-salt ratio. Per the kidneys' circadian rhythm, vasopressin increases around dinnertime so you don't produce as much urine at night. During the later third of the night, vasopressin spikes tell the body, "Hold your water!" so you don't wake up to pee. But if you get only six hours, that's two hours less of suppressed pee, so you lose more liquid during the day and are more likely to be dehydrated. In short, your body produces urine when it would otherwise conserve water.

Short sleepers pee more. They lose more water than those who get a full seven or eight hours.

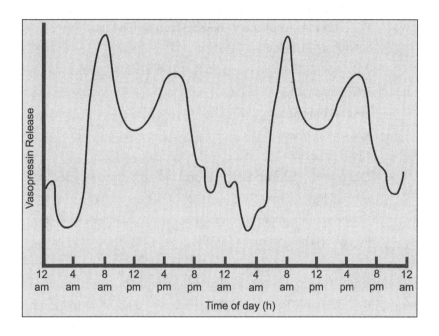

DRINKING PROBLEM #5:
MISTAKING BLOAT FOR HYDRATION

Bloating feels like you've been pumped full of gas and/or retained fluid. Bloat makes me think about videos I've seen of people injecting huge syringes of brine into their Thanksgiving turkey before roasting it. No one wants to feel like a swollen turkey. Due to hormonal shifts, premenstrual women can gain as much as six pounds of water weight before their periods. There's not much they can do about it, except supplement with vitamin B6[13] and eat foods high in fiber, magnesium, and potassium, such as bananas, avocados, melons, leafy greens, or brussels sprouts, for example. Pregnant women also experience leg swelling due to hormonal changes.

Other causes of water retention:

- **High-salt, high-carb foods**
- **Deficiencies in dietary magnesium and potassium**
- **Sedentary lifestyle**
- **Air travel** (Compression socks! Just try them. You can thank me later.)
- **Heart disease**
- **Kidney disease**
- **Liver disease**
- **Deep vein thrombosis**, a blood clot that causes edema in the legs. This condition is life-threatening. If you notice swelling, pain, warm skin, and tenderness in your leg, go to the ER immediately.

Logically, it might seem as if the best way to deal with water retention is to drink less. But that isn't how the body works. The counterintuitive strategy is far more effective. To ease symptoms of water retention, drink *more* water. The body retains fluid if the sodium level in your blood is high. It releases water when sodium is low. It's always trying to balance the water-salt ratio. One way to lower sodium (and release fluid) is to add more water. Another way is to eat potassium-rich foods such as bananas, avocados, spinach, sweet potatoes, and peaches. Sodium and potassium sit on opposite sides of a seesaw. Increase one, and the other falls.

Diuretics are substances that make you release water. Diuretic foods and beverages make you dump water *and* salt. A few servings of these will make anyone who's bloated (including women with PMS) feel much more comfortable:

- **High-dose caffeine**. Two cups won't do it. The third one, however, will have a diuretic effect.[14]

- **Coconut water** suppresses vasopressin. In a recent study, it had a greater diuretic effect than an actual diuretic when given to rats.[15]
- **Parsley.** This leafy herb is packed with vitamins A, C, and K, and antioxidant flavonoids and carotenoids. It's a superfood that also makes you pee.
- **Watermelon.** This water-rich fruit contains the antioxidant lycopene, vitamins A, B5, and C, potassium, and the heart-healthy amino acids L-arginine and citrulline. It's both hydrating *and* a diuretic.
- **Celery.** Fibrous celery is packed with diuretic minerals such as magnesium, potassium, and calcium, a perfect choice to nudge your floodgates open.

DRINKING PROBLEM #6: DRINKING UNFILTERED TAP WATER

Hydration is a hot topic in our rapidly warming climate. Along with anxiety about access to clean drinking water, people are becoming more aware of the chemicals and bacteria in the water supply and how they affect health.

Not all water is equal. Tap water might be contaminated with mold, pesticides, pharmaceutical drugs, heavy metals, and chemicals such as chlorine, which has been associated with increased colorectal cancer risk.[16]

You can check the quality of your tap water by typing in your ZIP code at the Environmental Working Group's Tap Water Database (find it at ewg.org/tapwater). When I did this, I discovered that the tap water in my California neighborhood contains thirty-two contaminants, including thirteen chemicals in excess of EWG's health guidelines. I had no idea.

When you do punch in your ZIP code and see what's in your water, the information will probably be both alarming and meaningless. What does it mean, for example, that your tap water has eighty times the healthy amount of bromodichloromethane? What is that? It says on the website that it can "potentially cause cancer." How potentially? If it's so deadly, how on earth is it coming through your tap?

Many of the chemicals tracked by EWG fall under the umbrella category of disinfectant byproducts (DBPs). Municipal water treatment facilities use these chemicals to clean the water supply of contaminants such as mold. That's good. But all chemical processes create byproducts, and the byproducts themselves are not always good. According to the Centers for Disease Control and Prevention, "Chronic exposure to DBPs may increase risk of cancer. Humans exposed to unusually large amounts of some DBPs could experience liver damage and decreased nervous system activity."[17] Studies have found that DBPs in tap water are "endocrine disrupting chemicals," which negatively affect fertility in both men and women.[18]

Two categories of DBPs to watch out for when you check your tap water:

- **Total trihalomethanes**, such as chloroform, bromoform, bromodichloromethane, and dibromochloromethane
- **Haloacetic acids**, such as monochloroacetic acid, dichloroacetic acid, trichloroacetic acid, and dibromoacetic acid

If you have tap water with high levels of contaminants such as DBPs, I hope you'll consider filtering your water, given the potential consequences of ingesting these chemicals, along with metals, dirt, and mold that might be in your home's plumbing. (I'll go into filtration systems in the next chapter.)

> ***Scary Water Wisdom***: *Not only should you know what's in your water, you should care about the vessel you use to drink from. A few years ago, the alarm went out about the danger of microplastics that wind up in the environment and your body. Even more insidious are nanoplastics. Per a 2024 study, there are 240,000 particles of nanoplastics in a liter-sized plastic bottle, accounting for 90 percent of all plastic particles in the bottle of water. The teeny-tiny molecules are more dangerous than their larger (but still bad) microplastic cousins because, in theory, nanoplastics are tiny enough to work their way into the bloodstream, the liver, and the brain.*[19] *It's too soon to know the extent of the damage they do. But in the meantime,* **don't drink or eat out of plastic containers when you can avoid doing so**.

Lots of *don'ts* in this chapter. I don't blame anyone from feeling the weight of all those *don'ts* and alarm about how to strike a healthy balance between over- and underhydration, between water and salt, between being a water zealot or stoic.

Coming up, I'm going to counterbalance all these *don'ts* with drinking *do's*.

TAKEAWAYS

- The whole-body health consequences of underhydration (being chronically low on fluid) and dehydration (an acute case of failing to replenish after a workout, for example) are huge: illness, inflammation, low energy, low blood pressure, poor physical and mental performance, headaches, constipation.

- Many people don't drink enough water because they don't want to stop for bathroom breaks, or they forget, or they have conditioned themselves to ignore thirst cues—all bad hydration habits that need to be changed.

- It is possible to overhydrate. When you drink too much water, the water-salt ratio is thrown off. In some cases, your brain swells and you could pass out, or worse.

- Bloating, or water retention, is caused by hormonal shifts, excessive salt intake, and inactivity. Counterintuitively, to decrease bloat, drink more water to right the water-salt ratio and cause the kidneys to dump excess fluid.

- We should be grateful that, in the U.S., we have readily available water out of the tap. However, our tap water can contain contaminants that negatively impact health and that can be filtered as needed. Plastic bottles shed micro- and nanoplastics into water, and should be avoided whenever possible. Just be aware that all water is not equal, or perfect.

CHAPTER 8

Drink for the Win

Six SIMPLE rules to get hydration down, and overall good health will flow into place.

DRINK DOMINO GOODIES

digestive glory
longer lifespan
longer healthspan
weight loss
reduced inflammation
sharper cognition
hot sex

TOP SIX SOLUTIONS FOR HEALTHY DRINKING

Know your need.
Establish a hydration habit.
Sip.
Enjoy with food.
Choose the good stuff.
Circulate.

A well-hydrated (but not oversaturated) body is a fount of good health. Some of the benefits that will flow into your life when you get drinking down:

Digestive glory. In a well-hydrated body, the colon doesn't have to suck water from food waste. Feces stay soft and slide effortlessly through the bowels. But that's not all hydration does for the digestive process. The colon is coated with two layers of gut-associated mucosal tissue (GALT). This mucus provides a slippery barrier between the colon wall and stool, protecting your bowel from injury.[1] The GALT is also home to the microbiome, the "world within" of trillions of cells of bacteria, fungi, and viruses that aids in digestion, immunity, and hormone production. Bringing it back to hydration, the gut mucus layers are 98 percent water,[2] and we produce 1 to 1.5 liters of mucus per day. That would not be possible without replenishing fluid loss. By meeting your hydration need and eating a diet of fiber- and water-rich fruits and vegetables,[3] you give your colon what it needs to maintain the all-important GALT.

Up your elimination game further by drinking mineral water from a natural source such as a mountain spring or glacier. For a recent study, German researchers divided their 106 functionally constipated participants into two groups: one that for six weeks drank up to 500 ml per day of natural mineral water high in sodium, magnesium, calcium, sulphate, and hydrogen carbonate, and another that drank the same amount of a placebo low-mineral water. For the duration of study, both groups recorded the frequency, ease, and consistency of their bowel movements, as well as their general sense of well-being. At the end (as it were), the group drinking water rich in minerals reported significant increases in spontaneous, completed bowel movements and improvement in stool consistency, compared to the control group. They also reported a higher quality of life after just six weeks of drinking mineral water. By making one tiny change — water choice — they were *so much happier.*[4]

Longer lifespan. Just think of it: By drinking, you'll have more years of glorious bowel elimination to enjoy! In a 2022 study, scientists in China found an association between hydration and long life by analyzing data on the dietary habits of 35,463 American adults over a fifteen-year period. Adequate water intake correlated with lower mortality risks from cancer and heart disease.[5] Simply put, in the U.S., there is evidence that drinking more water makes you less likely to die horribly from a terminal illness.

Longer healthspan. Living for a long time sounds great, but only if you're well enough to enjoy it. In 2022 research, the National Institutes of Health analyzed twenty-five years' worth of data from some 11,000 adults who were 45 to 66 at the start of the study and 70 to 90 at the end. They found that the well-hydrated subjects stayed in better health as they got older compared to their less hydrated counterparts. Researchers focused on two key factors: blood serum sodium (representing hydration habits) and biological age compared to chronological age (for speed of aging and disease risk). None of the participants' serum sodium was out of normal range, which is 135 to 146 mmol per liter. Those at the high end, at 144 mmol, had a greater risk of life-threatening diseases such as heart failure, stroke, diabetes, lung disease, and dementia, plus a 21 percent higher risk of all-cause mortality (dying for any reason). Those at 142 mmol were 50 percent more likely to have a higher biological age vs. chronological age than their less-salty counterparts.[6] The study's author, Natalia Dmitrieva, PhD, a researcher at the Laboratory of Cardiovascular Regenerative Medicine at the National Heart, Lung, and Blood Institute, told the NIH, "The results suggest that proper hydration may slow down aging and prolong a disease-free life."[7]

Hydration might not be the only reason subjects stayed sprightly and disease free as they got older. Researchers believe that the conscientious water drinkers made smarter choices in general, which preserved their youth and good health. As I've been saying all along, get the drink domino down, and other good habits will follow.

Weight loss. I want to quickly dispense the myth that drinking a ton will fool the stomach into thinking it's full, thereby decreasing appetite. It takes about ten minutes for fluid to exit the stomach. Once it has passed into the small intestine, the stomach is no longer full, and will start grumbling again. If anything, this strategy only *delays* hunger briefly. Of course, if you do get hungry (or tungry) between meals, it's a good idea to drink a glass of water instead of eating a high-sugar, high-fat snack. Or, even better, have a high-protein snack with a glass of water to speed up metabolism, hydrate, and ward off carb cravings all at the same time.

Not a myth: Drink water before a meal to eat less food. Science bears this out. For older overweight or obese adults who struggle to lose weight, drinking a pint of water before breakfast *does* help you eat significantly fewer calories.[8] In another study, researchers in Mumbai, India, had fifty overweight women drink 500 ml (about 16 ounces) of water a half-hour before breakfast, lunch, and dinner every day for eight weeks. These servings were above and beyond their normal water consumption. Their weight, body mass index (BMI), and body-fat percentage were taken before and after the study period. Just from making that one change in their drinking habits, the subjects' BMI, weight, and body fat decreased significantly. The researchers concluded that water before a meal ignited thermogenesis, or the body using stored fat as fuel to maintain body temperature.[9]

Water Wisdom: You can burn more calories by drinking water before a meal in a process called water-induced thermogenesis. A German study found that drinking 16 ounces of room-temperature water increased energy expenditure (how much fuel the body uses) by 30 percent. The faster-burn effect lasted only about forty minutes,[10] so you're not going to drop a lot of weight via water-induced thermogenesis. But every little boost of energy expenditure helps.

Reduced inflammation. Here's a lightning-fast course on one way that inflammation happens: Unstable atoms called free radicals are the byproduct of breathing. Since we all draw breath, we all have free radicals floating around the body. Ordinarily, this is no big deal. The immune system patrols for them, hunts them down, and neutralizes them. Antioxidants render them harmless. However, if free radicals are not eradicated or neutralized, they can damage DNA and cause a tumor to grow. When they proliferate, they cause oxidative stress. (Oxidation is the same process that causes iron to rust.) The immune system responds to free radicals by sending an army of defender cells. All good and healthy. That's the body doing what it's designed to do. But, if oxidative stress is chronic, the immune response becomes chronic, too. White blood cells rush to the site of oxidative stress and just stay there, inflaming the area. Chronic inflammation is a major problem that can lead to arthritis, diabetes, heart disease, stroke, and dementia.

Drinking water is an excellent preventative of oxidative stress and the inflammation it causes. Hydration helps maintain a beneficial ratio of free radicals (oxidants) to antioxidants, ensuring that the unstable atoms can do you no harm. The anti-inflammatory hydration benefit was discovered to be especially meaningful during exercise recovery.[11] So after a workout, replenish fluids and visualize every drop washing your insides clean of free radicals and oxidative stress.

Sharper cognition. I can't say hydration will make you smarter. Your intellect is what it is. But sufficient hydration can improve memory and concentration. A classic British study[12] from 2012 looked at 447 psychology students at the University of East London who went into an exam hall to take a big test. Twenty-five percent of them happened to bring water into the exam with them. Those who did scored on average 5 percent higher marks compared to their dry-mouthed counterparts. (The researchers controlled for academic ability.) The lead researcher believed that, in addition to increasing concentration, taking sips helped the students allieviate their anxiety during the test. If drinking water can buy you half a grade, or give you an edge at work, or help you concentrate while playing Wordle, that seems worth it to me.

Hot sex. Sex and fluids. There is definitely a connection.

As I've heard, the most important sex organ is the one between your ears: your brain. I'm not going to debate whether that's true. But I can tell you that the brain is about 75 percent water, and if it's shrunken due to dehydration, it will not be up for a quickie, or a longie. A well-documented symptom of mild dehyration is a headache,[13] which has become such a common reason for partners to beg off sex that it's a cliché ("Not tonight, dear, I have a headache").

Now, about those other sexual organs.

Erectile dysfuction is usually a blood flow issue. And when you are dehydrated, you have lower blood volume and increased blood pressure. On hydraulics alone, it is harder (irony alert) to get an erection when dehydrated. If you are hydrated, erection strength and speed get a big lift (as it were).

Regarding female parts, the clitoris is made of erectile tissue that requires blood flow and hydration for proper functioning. Women have Skene's glands tucked up in the vulva that have the sole purpose of secreting fluid to lubricate the area when stimulated. Vulva-vaginal fluid is 90 percent water. It protects delicate skin from chafing, itching, and tearing and therefore decreases the risk of infection. Vaginal dryness is, in part, a hydration issue. When a woman is dehydrated, the body reroutes precious fluid toward vital organs to keep her alive, and away from joints, tissues, and skin. You could say that, when sexually aroused, the vulva and vagina are *the most* vital organs. But the body will send fluid to the brain instead.

And one more thing: UTIs can occur when bacteria is introduced to the urethal opening during sexual activity. The best defense against infection is to urinate after sex. The stream washes the bacteria out of the urinary tract. Just another good reason for women to drink a glass of water in anticipation of having sex.

⸙

So much to gain, just from doing something as simple as taking a refreshing drink of clean, clear water. I'll make the practice even easier for you. Here are the Top Six Solutions for Healthy Drinking:

DRINK SOLUTION #1: KNOW YOUR NEED

According to the Centers for Disease Control, on average, adults in the U.S. drink 43 ounces of plain water per day. None of the dozens of studies I read have found that that amount is nearly enough. But there's debate within the hydration community about what people should aim for.

The best-known benchmark is 64 ounces per day (eight 8-ounce servings).

Other experts believe that healthy adults who are not suffering from heart or kidney disease should drink half an ounce for every pound of weight, so a 150-pound woman should consume 75 ounces of water per day.

Kardashians and social media influencers encourage their followers to buy $45 40-ounce stainless steel Stanley cups (my daughter has one with her name on it) and promise glowing skin if they drink a gallon per day. That's 128 ounces.

One study by doctors with the U.S. Army Research Institute of Environmental Medicine recommends a baseline of 125 ounces for men and 91 ounces for women per day.[14]

The National Academy of Medicine's guideline is thirteen 8-ounce cups a day for men and nine cups for women.

Other experts advise that you drink 8 ounces of water each hour for the first ten hours per day after waking, or 80 ounces total.

If people work out, they need to factor that into the equation. Per the "Galpin Equation," you should drink your body weight in pounds divided by 30 for every fifteen minutes of exercise. For a 150-pound woman, the formula is: 150/30 = 5 ounces. If she exercises for an hour, she needs to add 20 ounces (5 x 4 = 20) to her daily total.

Given all this discussion, one thing is abundantly clear:

There is no universally accepted calculation for water need.

When I created my own formula, I took another factor into account: "turnover rate," or the speed at which water moves through the body, from lips to bowl. Do you pee very quickly after drinking? Do you retain fluid? According to a 2022 Japanese study of over 5,000 people from all over the world, individual variations of turnover rates are huge. Ranges vary widely from person to person and region to region.[15] Generally, for men in their twenties and women in their twenties, thirties, and forties, turnover rate is rapid. Those age groups need to replenish more because of that fast turnover.

Other factors to consider when estimating water need:

- **Age**. Tweens are fine with around 60 ounces per day; teens need around 75 ounces; adults need at least 80 ounces.
- **Weight**. The bigger you are, the more water you need to maintain blood volume.
- **Sex**. Men might have as much as a 25 percent greater water need than women.
- **Activity level**. Exercisers and athletes, especially those who sweat copiously, require more hydration than sedentary folks.

- **Location.** Do you live in a hot, dry climate or a cool, humid one? Hot and humid means more sweat, and therefore more water need. Altitude matters, too. People who live in low countries need to drink more than those at higher altitudes.
- **Medical issues.** If you are on prescription medication and/or have kidney disease, heart disease, or diabetes, consult your doctor about hydration needs.
- **Pregnancy and breastfeeding.** If you are pregnant, add 16 ounces to daily intake. Breastfeeding requires an extra liter per day.
- **Illness.** If you have a cold, the flu, kidney stones, are vomiting, or have diarrhea, increase intake along with electrolytes.
- **Diet.** Is your diet high in water-rich fruits and vegetables, or do you eat mostly dry foods like bread, crackers, beef jerky, and raisins? The more water rich your food, the less fluid you need to drink.

There is no cookie-cutter answer for the question "How much should I drink?" But since we need some kind of benchmark, I recommend this calculation for a spring, fall, or winter day:

(Weight in pounds x 0.6) + 12 oz. per thirty minutes of exercise = Daily intake in ounces

For a 150-pound woman who works out for one hour per day: (150 x 0.6) + 24 = 114

On a non-workout day: (150 x 0.6) + 0 = 90

During hot summer days, add 16 ounces.
So in August on leg day: (150 x 0.6) + 24 + 16 = 130

If you don't want to make yourself crazy with formulas—I do NOT blame you—you can just make sure you drink 16 ounces of water—a pint-sized glass—five times per day. You can obviously drink at will at any other time. But if you commit to drinking five times per day, you will hit your water need.

In the Sleep-Drink-Breathe Plan (coming up later in the book), I recommend these five times:

1. Upon waking
2. Mid-morning
3. Lunchtime
4. A half-hour before dinner
5. Two hours before bedtime

The hydration-forgetful might be wondering how you're supposed to remember to drink at those times. I recommend you set alarms on your phone or watch. But even better . . .

DRINK SOLUTION #2: ESTABLISH A HYDRATION HABIT

According to a 2021 study by researchers at the University of Glasgow in Scotland, the key to making hydration a habit is feeling like it's a reward.[16] If the behavior comes with a reward of some kind—pleasure, pride, accomplishment—you will want to repeat it and cement it into your routine. But as their subjects told the Glasgow team, water just isn't as pleasurable as other beverages. Coffee is certainly pleasurable. If it weren't, it wouldn't be a globally treasured commodity, like chocolate. Drinking water, however refreshing, doesn't have the same reward system of flavor and caffeine built into it.

As you establish a hydration habit, just be aware going in that the reward is hydration itself, how good it makes you feel, and the knowledge of how beneficial it is for you. Personally, I have been a water guy for so long that I have trained myself to prefer the taste of water over other beverages.

Regardless of taste, you can make water feel like a reward if you tie it to another pleasurable behavior that's already an established habit. The good feelings associated with that behavior will spill into water drinking (this is called classical conditioning).

A friend of mine, a successful professional with a busy career and demanding family life, suffered from chronic underhydration. She would forget to drink and realize at dinnertime that she'd barely had a glass of anything since her morning coffee. I worked with her on some circadian-related issues and encouraged her to drink water upon waking, to substitute her morning coffee with herbal tea, and to have coffee at lunchtime instead. The idea was to get her to drink 16 to 24 ounces in the first two hours of the day. She accomplished that, but she was still falling short of her target of 90 ounces per day.

The hurdle was a lack of pleasure. She found drinking water tedious.

I asked, "What do you enjoy doing? What are your pleasures in life?"

She listed several things, like reading and spending time with her kids. "And evening TV. After dinner is all cleaned up and I've replied to any late-breaking work emails, I love settling into the couch and watching TV for a few hours."

I suggested that she make a pot of herbal tea before she hit the couch, and to sip steadily for the first hour of her viewing time. She tried it and loved it. She named her new evening ritual "tea and TV." Before long, she didn't have to remind herself to put on the kettle. This now became the automatic precursor to her watch party of one. By linking a pleasurable activity with hydration, she effort-lessly and joyfully gained 20 ounces of intake.

My buddy BJ Fogg, author of *Tiny Habits: The Small Changes That Change Everything*, says it takes about twenty-eight days to establish a new habit. A few years ago, I established a hydration habit that was part of a morning routine I called 3x15. Every morning upon wak-ing, I drink 15 ounces of water, get 15 minutes of sunlight (to rein-force my circadian rhythm), and take 15 belly breaths. I established this routine in just four weeks of daily commitment, until I stopped needing to remind myself to do them. Now I automatically reach for my room-temperature water, take it into my backyard, and sip while breathing deeply, often with my shoes off and feet in the grass. On the rare day that I can't follow the 3x15 morning routine, I miss it dearly. The entire day feels off. But as soon as I pick it back up the next morning, all is right in my world again. I just feel energized and prepared for the day — and whatever stressors that come with it.

Curveballs don't stop flying at you, even if you remember to hydrate. Life will still be full of stress. But if you have a healthy, habitual routine, you've trained for the pressure.

Do the work of creating a hydration habit now! Don't wait until you're past middle age. For seniors, mild dehydration is particularly worrisome because as we age, the thirst center signals grow weak. Seniors can't rely on thirst to remember to drink.[17]

HYDRATION MULTIPLIERS: HELP OR HYPE?

A hot hydration trend: "Hydration multipliers" are electroyte pow-ders you add to plain water. Online, they go for around $2 or more per serving. The name implies that the multipliers make water more hydrating than it would be without, that by adding electrolytes (sodium, potassium, magnesium, chloride, phosphate, and calcium), your body absorbs the fluid with more efficiency. Why drink three bottles of water if you can drink one, plus a packet of powder, for equal hydration?

It sounds great in theory. But do hydration multipliers live up to the promise?

If the goal is to absorb fluid more rapidly, the results are dubious and hard to measure.

Multiplier powders contain as much as 500+ mgs of sodium per dose, which is a lot for anyone who liberally seasons their food. It's a lot if you have kidney disease or take meds for high blood pressure. Per the Food and Drug Administration, the recommended daily allowance of sodium for adults is 2,300 mgs; on average, Americans consume 3,400 mgs.[18] So if you use more than one packet of powder per day — increasing sodium by 1,000+ mgs on top of what you already consume — you could push yourself into hypernatremia (too salty!) and experience diarrhea, dizziness, and nausea.

Some products contain as much as 11 grams of sugar, which isn't as bad as Gatorade, but it's not great. If you're prediabetic, diabetic, or insulin resistant, make sure your choice of powder is sugar free.

There is some evidence that taking electrolyte powder with water before or after a workout does help with recovery and maintenance of sodium levels.[19] Of course, you could just mix ⅛ teaspoon of salt (300 mgs of sodium) into a glass of water with a squirt of fresh-squeezed lemon and get the same result for pennies. Regarding the claim of a post-exercise recovery boost, eating a banana is just as beneficial as an electrolyte solution[20] and cheaper.

I'm not convinced that hydration multipliers are worth the cost when there are far less expensive alternatives. For convenience, however, it might be worth it to have a box in your medicine cabinet to use in specific circumstances, such as:

- **Extreme exercise.** I'm not talking about a three-mile jog. I mean a ten-mile, competitively paced run, or three hours of intense sports.
- **Extreme heat.** In 100-degree weather with no access to air conditioning, you will sweat significantly and rapidly. Lost fluid and salt needs to be replaced with an electrolyte-infused beverage.
- **Extreme sickness.** If you have gastritis or any condition that makes you vomit or have diarrhea for more than several hours, drinking an electrolyte solution, Pedialyte, or sugar-free Gatorade will help replace lost minerals.

HEAD-TO-HEAD: HYDRATION MULTIPLIERS

Comparison shopping of three popular brands online:

Liquid I.V. $24/16 packets ($1.50 each)	Primal Hydration $44/30 packets ($1.47 each)	LMNT $27/16 packets ($1.69 each)
Calories: 45	Calories: 7	Calories: 10
Carbs: 11 g	Carbs: 1.6 g	Carbs: 2 g
Sodium: 510 mg	Sodium: 400 mg	Sodium: 1,000 mg
Potassium: 380 mg	Potassium: 350 mg	Potassium: 200 mg
Magnesium: 0 mg	Magnesium: 50 mg	Magnesium: 60 mg
Zinc: 0 mg	Zinc: 0 mg	Zinc: 0 mg
Vitamin C: 76 mg	Vitamin C: 200 mg	Vitamin C: 0 mg
Niacin: 22.8 mg	Niacin: 20 mg	Niacin: 0 mg
Vitamin B6: 6.8 mg	Vitamin B6: 2 mg	Vitamin B6: 0 mg
Vitamin B12: 6.8 mcg	Vitamin B12: 20 mcg	Vitamin B12: 0 mcg

DRINK SOLUTION #3:
SIP

As previously mentioned, you have sensors in your mouth and throat that tell the brain "fluid incoming." After a minute of continuous drinking, the brain tells you, "Okay, that's enough. Stop drinking now." If you continued chugging after the cutoff signal, the body has a mechanism in place to protect you from the dangers of overhydration. Your kidneys respond to a deluge by kicking into overdrive and dumping fluid via urine.

> ***Water Wisdom***: *Drinking a large quantity of fluid – 20 or more ounces a few times a day – to hit your minimum is a bad hydration strategy. You'll just pee it out before it's had a chance to be absorbed and used by tissues and organs. Sipping is the real secret to hydration multiplying.*

Picture a kitchen sponge again. If you held it under a faucet at full blast, the sponge would quickly become oversaturated, and the water would just run off and swirl down the drain.

Hold the sponge under a trickle of water, and it will catch and absorb the fluid, stay wet, and take much longer to reach saturation. So when I say drink 15 ounces of water upon waking, I don't mean that I pound it back in four greedy gulps. It's best to sip an ounce (one swallow) at a time. It won't take more than several minutes to finish the glass. But by slowing down, you'll retain the fluid and use it.

DRINK SOLUTION #4:
ENJOY WITH FOOD

Eating + drinking is a great way to link a pleasurable behavior with hydration and help you establish hydration habits at three or more times per day. A few myths to bust about drinking water with food:

- **It makes you bloat.** Nope. Drinking water with a meal helps break food down into smaller, easier-to-digest morsels, *decreasing* the potential for bloating.
- **It interferes with digestion.** Also wrong. There is *already* water in your stomach, along with gastric acid and enzymes. They all work together to turn food into mush. A glass of water will not dilute the acid in your stomach or slow food breakdown. Think about it logically: Soups, stews, fruits, vegetables—all water-rich foods—are considered among the healthiest options out there.
- **It hinders nutrient absorption.** Vitamins, minerals, proteins, carbs, and fats are not absorbed in the stomach. That process takes place in the small intestine. By the time food gets there, it's been turned into slurry, thanks in part to water. Slurry is the ideal consistency to pass through the guts, where the cilia that line the small intestine walls reach out and grab nutrients to absorb and pass into the bloodstream.
- **Drinking with food is less hydrating than water alone.** False! Combining protein and fats with fluids aids in the absorption of the most essential nutrient of all: water.

FOUNTAIN OF YOUTH FOODS

Up to 20 percent of your water intake comes from food. Eating a plant-based, water-rich diet (for example, a Mediterranean diet)—loads of veggies, fruit, seeds, nuts, and lean protein—lengthens telomeres, the little end caps on DNA strands that shrink with age, per a 2019 study.[21] You don't have to go full vegan. Just by having an extra salad or apple, you sneak in additional hydration, along with vitamins, minerals, and antioxidants that keep you healthy. Want an easy trick to determine whether you're eating a fiber-rich diet? A nutritionist once told me, "Water- and fiber-rich whole foods retain their shape if you run them under water." I think about that all the time and choose whole foods that hold their own.

According to the USDA National Nutrient Database,[22] here's the water content of some foods:

- 90–99% water: cantaloupe, strawberries, watermelon, lettuce, cabbage, celery, spinach, pickles, squash, asparagus, tomato, cauliflower, lettuce, mushrooms, peppers, pumpkin
- 80–89% water: yogurt, apples, blueberries, grapes, citrus fruit, cherries, kiwi, mango, peach, plum, carrots, broccoli, pears, pineapple, green beans, brussels sprouts, onions
- 70–79% water: bananas, avocados, cottage cheese, ricotta, potato, corn, shrimp
- 60–69% water: pasta, legumes, salmon, chicken
- 50–59% water: beef, hot dogs, feta cheese
- 40–49% water: pizza
- 30–39% water: hard cheese, bread
- 20–29% water: sausage, cake
- 10–19% water: butter, dried fruit
- 1–9% water: nuts, peanut butter, cookies, crackers, dry cereal
- 0% water: oil, sugar

DRINK SOLUTION #5:
CHOOSE THE GOOD STUFF

Which water—mineral, spring, tap, or purified—is most hydrating? In descending order:

Mineral water. The Federal Drug Administration has clear guidelines for a product to be labeled mineral water. It has to contain "not less than 250 parts per million total dissolved solids [minerals and trace elements]" and come from a "geologically and physically protected underground water source" that most likely runs over rocks where it picks up all those goodies.[23] The minerals—calcium, magnesium, potassium, sodium, bicarbonate, zinc, and iron, among others—have to be naturally occurring and come from the source. All that magnesium helps lower blood pressure and serves as a digestive aid. The calcium strengthens bones.

> **Water Wisdom**: You can make mineral water at home. An easy recipe:
>
> Filter one liter or quart of tap water. In order, add ⅛ teaspoon of baking soda, ⅛ teaspoon of Epsom salt, ⅛ teaspoon of potassium bicarbonate. Then mix it well. Or you can buy combined trace minerals in liquid form online or at a GNC and just squeeze a dropperful into a glass of drinking water.

Spring water. To earn an FDA label of "spring" water, the liquid had to come from a natural source, too, but it doesn't necessarily run over rocks and pick up as many (or *any*) minerals. Spring water often does contain some magnesium, calcium, potassium, and sodium. About 60 percent of tap water comes from the same sources as spring water. However ...

Tap water has been chemically scrubbed of contaminants (but not perfectly, as previously discussed) and is just as "clean" as spring water. The benefit of using tap is that you won't add to the 500 billion plastic bottles per year that are polluting the planet. Just fill your own stainless steel or glass bottle with tap water at home and, if needed, filter it with an activated carbon filter (which won't filter out minerals).

Pure or distilled water has been intentionally depleted of minerals. Marketers label it as "pure," and it is—pure crap. I call it "empty water." If you were to drink nothing but purified water, your body would have a net loss of minerals because stores of them would be swept out in urine. The best use for pure or distilled water is in your humidifier, neti pot, or CPAP machine. But don't bother drinking it.

Now, about filtration. I do recommend that you get some kind of filter for tap water that will pay for itself quickly enough when you stop buying bottled water. There are hundreds, if not thousands, of options for at-home water filtration systems. Big name brands in this space are PUR and Brita, but there are dozens more available online or at any hardware or home goods store. The prices range from $20 to thousands. Many new refrigerators come with water filter systems pre-installed. They are okay at removing contaminants, but you have to replace the filter every six months, which people tend to forget to do. They are also not as effective as the systems listed below. But, honestly, any filtration is better than none.

The pros and cons of various units:

Under-the-Counter Filters

Pros: They are permanent installations. One you get it in there, with a separate faucet for just filtered water, you don't have to worry about it again, apart from regularly changing the filter. It does a thorough job of filtering chemicals and contaminants and makes your water taste great.

Cons: It's complicated to set up, with a bunch of hoses and possible drilling into your countertop, so most people need to factor in the cost of hiring someone to install it. Units start in the hundreds, and the replacement filters aren't cheap either.

Faucet-Mounted Filters

Pros: They do an excellent job of eliminating chemicals and contaminants and make water chef-kiss delicious. The installation is far less complicated than an under-the-sink unit, but if you're not DIY inclined, it might be worth it to have a Task Rabbit helper do it for you, just to be sure it's on right. The price is under $50, with replacement filters running around $25.

Cons: It takes up space in the sink area, which can be annoying. Some might not find these units to be aesthetically pleasing. If they're not properly installed, water may spurt all over the place.

Countertop Filters

Pros: They're small and portable. You could even travel with one, if you take a vacation and want to have filtered water at the lake house. They're highly effective at removing unwanted substances and give you clear water that tastes clean. In terms of ease of use, they're sort of like coffee makers, ready to go, right out of the box.

Cons: Also like a coffee maker, they take up precious counter space and aren't exactly stunning to behold. You can filter only a carafe of water at time. And they're pricey, some units costing $500 or more, plus replacement filters.

Pitchers

Pros: Inexpensive! They start at $20, with replacement filters around the same price. Efficient! They're just as good at clearing contaminants as the pricey units. Cute! Some pitchers are quite aesthetically pleasing, and they hold a good volume of water, too.

Cons: I have found that a pitcher lasts about as long as a toaster. After a year or two of daily use, something breaks and it has to be replaced. But at that cost, it doesn't hurt much.

#WATERTRENDS

Do any of them make a difference in terms of hydration? Glad you asked:

Alkaline water has been ionized and filtered to have a pH number in the 8 or 9 range (neutral is 7; coffee is 4.8 to 5.5). The idea is that if you drink alkaline water, you will neutralize acid in the blood that purportedly causes all kinds of problems. But there isn't much research that says alkaline water cures disease or aids digestion. The kidneys naturally balance pH in the body—keeping it at a slightly basic 7.4—regardless of what you eat and drink, so by drinking alkaline water, you're causing the body to work harder to maintain its ideal pH and use energy it could better spend in other ways.

Hydrogen water is plain water, plus extra molecules of hydrogen gas. You can buy hydrogen water in bottles or get tablets to drop into bottled water. The hype is that extra hydrogen makes water anti-inflammatory, anti-aging, and energizing. There is some truth to the hype. Hydrogen water has been found to reduce LDL ("bad") cholesterol and inflammatory markers.[24] It might quiet the sympathetic nervous system, which means less stress and higher quality of life.[25] A 2021 study tested thirty-seven volunteers on the effects of hydrogen water to see if it improved athletic performance and reduced fatigue. Half of the participants were trained cyclists; the other half were just normal people. Some took a placebo for a week; the rest drank hydrogen water for the same length of time. At the end of the trial, only one group saw an increase in power and decrease in fatigue: the cyclists who drank the hydrogen water. So it did work, but only by improving athletic performance while training.[26]

Carbonated water. Seltzer + alcohol, the hot trend of…always. Hey, White Claw, ever heard of a wine spritzer? You know that alcohol interferes with vasopressin and is a net-zero hydration option. So stick with sugar-free seltzer minus the booze. A myth I've heard for years is that water with pressurized carbon dioxide bubbles tastes great but is not as thirst quenching or hydrating. Not true. Ounce per ounce, seltzer is just as hydrating as flat water, and, for my money, it's refreshing, especially with a slice of lime.

DRINK SOLUTION #6: CIRCULATE

One thing that doesn't come up often enough is the partnership between hydration and movement. If you are sedentary, gravity draws fluids down to where your butt hits the couch. If you sit for hours at a time, your vessels get constricted, narrowing the space for blood and lymph to flow. The worst-case scenario is dehydration combined with fluid stagnation, with resulting swelling, bloating, and toxin buildup. Even if you're well hydrated, you still need to boost circulation with movement to (1) carry nutrients and oxygen to cells and (2) sweep up toxins for elimination in urine. Being hydrated and sedentary is like having a full cup of water with a thick layer of sludge on the bottom. It's just going to stay there unless you shake it up and filter it.

When you're active, your heart rate increases and your bloodstream picks up speed, sweeps up body sludge, and takes it to the liver and kidneys to be filtered and eliminated. Hydration/detox tip: You can use water outside your body to invigorate the movement of fluid inside your body by alternating between hot and cold showers.

Perspiration revs up your body's hydration regulatory system. When you break a sweat, your thirst command center notices the dip in your blood sodium concentration and sends a loud message to your brain, "Water needed, stat!" As long as you replace the fluid and electrolytes lost to sweat (in addition to your daily drink need), you will stimulate circulation and aid your body's detoxification process. You don't even have to work out. You can schvitz in a steam room, sauna, or infrared blanket.

But you don't have to sweat to circulate. Just getting up from your computer periodically to get a fresh glass of water can be a great way to habit-stack and get hydration and circulation at the same time.

So now that you know all about how to keep good health afloat by sleeping and drinking, it's time to make a pot of tea, take a deep breath, and get ready to learn about the third Domino of Wellness.

TAKEAWAYS

- A well-hydrated body does everything better: digesting, thinking, circulating blood and lymphatic fluid, detoxing, having sex, and exercising.
- Drinking water is the fountain of youth. The well hydrated fend off disease and live longer than others.
- Drinking room-temperature water a half-hour before meals makes you eat less and burn more fat.
- Your hydration needs depend on several factors, including age, weight, activity level, location, and sex. But you can calculate your water goal with a simple

formula: (**Weight in pounds x 0.6**) + **12 oz. per thirty minutes of exercise = Daily intake in ounces.** Or just drink one 8-ounce glass of water for each of the first ten waking hours per day.

- For maximum absorption, sip, don't chug.
- The best quality water in order: mineral, spring, filtered tap. Not "pure" or distilled. The best vessel for drinking: stainless steel, glass, ceramic. Not plastic!
- If you eat water- and fiber-rich foods (fruits and veggies, mainly), you can boost your hydration in the most delicious way.
- Move your body to rev up circulation. Hydration and good circulation work together to nourish cells, support functions, and detox your whole body.

DOMINO THREE

breathe

Simplify health and wellness by getting
the third fundamental biobehavior down.

CHAPTER 9

Breathe 411

Inspirational facts about something you do up to
20,000 times a day

WHAT IS BREATHING?

WHY DO YOU NEED TO BREATHE?

WHAT HAPPENS WHEN YOU TAKE A BREATH?

HOW DOES NOT BREATHING KILL YOU?

Everyone knows that working out can greatly reduce stress, increase energy, or be an important outlet for pent-up emotion. And we're all for sweating it out to a better outlook. But before you shell out for the expensive group fitness class—or turn to a sugary sweet to beat the 3:00 p.m. slump—did you know that simple breathing techniques you can start right this minute can offer the same release as a workout, reenergize you through the afternoon doldrums, and even increase brain power and improve sleep? Best part—they are completely, utterly free.

Of the three Dominos of Wellness, breathing is the most overlooked. Even five years ago, the mainstream media rarely, if ever, blasted headlines about the dangers of breathing incorrectly. Even now, I doubt there will be a #breathchallenge on TikTok that showcases close-up videos of a creator's nostrils. Yoga people, however, have been aware of the incredible healing, stimulating, and calming powers of breath for millennia. What's really catching on are breathing workshops. They are becoming super popular in the wellness community—with good reason. It matters how you draw air in and out of your lungs. That understanding is finally reaching critical mass. And I am here for it. I've been focused on breathing techniques—as a sleep doctor, in a group setting, and in my individual practice—for many years, and have a ton of fascinating stuff to share with you about it.

WHAT IS BREATHING?

When we inhale, we draw oxygen and nitrogen from the atmosphere into the nose and mouth.

When we exhale, we send carbon dioxide and nitrogen out through the nose and mouth into the atmosphere.

That two-part process, the cycle of inhalation and exhalation, is what "taking a breath" means. You can't have inhalation without exhalation because both are essential to staying alive.

WHY DO YOU NEED TO BREATHE?

In the simplest terms, we breathe to turn glucose into energy so we can function.

The step-by-step of cellular respiration: Inside your body, you have stores of sugar (glycogen, made from glucose). Glucose comes from food and is stashed for later use in the liver, muscles, and other places. Picture those glucose units as little sugar cubes. When you take a breath, the incoming oxygen (O_2) acts like a lit match that, when it comes into contact with those sugar cubes, sets them on fire. The heat generated from the fire is energy that maintains body temperature and powers the body's fifteen trillion cells. Brain cells use energy to think, remember, concentrate, and to tell our systems what to do and when. Heart cells use energy to pump blood. Muscle cells use it to run, type, dance, and breathe. Without oxygen, the entire process of turning glucose into fuel would not have its spark.

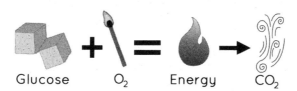

Glucose O_2 Energy CO_2

Keeping the visual going, a burning sugar cube produces heat and smoke. Smoke is the byproduct of the chemical reaction that creates energy. In this metaphor, smoke is carbon dioxide (CO_2), the waste product of cellular respiration. CO_2 has a bad reputation because we associate it with the toxic smog belching from car exhaust pipes and factory smokestacks. But the gas isn't *all* bad, just as O_2 isn't all good. Once again, it's about homeostasis, balance.

> ***Water Wisdom + Air Awareness***: With hydration,
> the essential balance is between water and salt.
> With breathing, the essential balance is between
> CO_2 and O_2 gasses.

So what does CO_2 do for you?

For starters, it regulates blood pH, keeping it at the optimal ever-so-slightly alkaline 7.4 pH, preventing that number from sliding into the acidic end of the scale.[1]

Carbon dioxide tweaks the shape of hundreds of millions of hemoglobin molecules (the protein in red blood cells responsible for transporting gasses throughout the body) to turn them into little buckets, so much the better to carry O_2 wherever it needs to go.[2]

Without CO_2, the "respiration drive" would be stalled. Like "sleep drive," a gradual buildup of chemicals in the brain that makes you feel increasingly tired (adenosine), respiration drive is a buildup of *pressure* to draw breath. As soon as the CO_2 to O_2 ratio in the blood tilts toward too much CO_2, the brain sends a signal to the respiration system that says, "Inhale *now*."

The sleep drive builds slowly over the course of the day, and you kind of know it's happening because you get sleepier and start yawning.

The respiration drive happens up to 20,000 times a day, usually without your being aware of it. It's like a tiny drama, a somewhat tense conversation between the head and the lungs, that always ends the same way, with an inhalation. Followed by an exhalation. And so on, and on, until death.

WHAT HAPPENS WHEN YOU TAKE A BREATH?

The incredible journey of an oxygen molecule begins in the atmosphere, the mixture of gasses, aka air, that hovers around the Earth thanks to gravity. You can't really see air or feel it, but you are moving through it every second of every day. The invisible stuff that surrounds you is made of 21 percent O_2, 78 percent nitrogen, and 1 percent other gasses, including CO_2, argon, and methane.

When the medulla oblongata, in the brain stem — part of the "lizard brain" that controls involuntary biobehaviors like breathing and digestion — senses that the balance of O_2 and CO_2 is off, it sends a message to the diaphragm, the dome-shaped muscle in the abdomen, right under the lungs, to flatten. That action makes the lungs expand, creating a vacuum that forces air into the nose and mouth, a process called inspiration. (Not just for artists!)

If you don't inhale when the respiration drive tells you to, you start to feel "air hunger," a gnawing sensation of deep need that's similar to intense food hunger. The symptoms of air hunger: a burning, tight chest; dizziness; the increasingly desperate urge to breathe. If you ignore these cues and willfully hold your breath until you pass out, your lungs will start breathing again for you automatically.

I was crazy enough to give a lecture and go through an Extreme Performance Training weekend (XPT) with Laird Hamilton (GOAT of surfing) and his wife, Gabby Reece (GOAT of Olympian beach volleyball), at their home in Malibu. Along with about thirty other loonies, I went through three days of extreme training (they kept us very well hydrated and fed). The pool work was the most interesting. When Gabby says jump, you do what she says, so I jumped into the pool and grabbed a 25-pound dumbbell. She said, "Blow all your air out and when you get to the bottom, walk all the way across the pool, put the dumbbell down gently, and then surface for air." When you are under water, holding 25 pounds, and Laird tells you, just before you get in, "Don't you ever drop the weights in the pool; they can crack the bottom," there are two types of pressure on you. And it does not take long for the air hunger to arrive.

During inhalation, aka inspiration, humans draw in sextillions of atoms of gasses, along with dust, dirt, pollutants, allergens, bacteria, mold, viruses. Unless you live on top of a mountain surrounded by tall pines, air is far from pure or clean. Fortunately, the body has a system in place to filter each breath so that many of the toxic bits don't cause harm. The nasal passages are lined with two layers of mucus that catch most of the pathogens and pollutants. Our mouths and throats are also coated with mucus, but those layers don't do as good a job of trapping germs and allergens as nasal mucus. It's just one of several reasons to inhale through the nose whenever possible (more on that later).

The inhaled molecules are heated, moistened, and concentrated as they flow through the sinuses and into the trachea, aka the windpipe. The trachea is an upside-down Y, branching into bronchi that lead directly into the right and left lungs. The bronchi split again and again into smaller bronchioles. The airway system looks like an inverted tree, with the windpipe as the trunk, the bronchi as large branches, and the bronchioles as smaller boughs. The surface area of your airways is also lined with mucus. The word *mucus* can be a turnoff, I know. But if it weren't for the goo, your lungs would be extremely vulnerable to bacteria and respiratory illnesses. Plus, if your lungs weren't lubricated, every exhalation — and the accompanying vapor loss at the rate of 17 ml per hour — would cause severe dehydration.

At the end of each bronchiole are clusters of microscopic structures that look like grapes, called alveoli. The 480 million alveoli are air sacs, like tiny balloons, covered with a lattice of capillaries. Oxygen molecules get sucked all the way into the air sacs, and from there, they migrate across the alveoli's walls and into nearby capillaries. Once an O_2 molecule enters the bloodstream, it hitches a ride on a red blood cell and is transported somewhere in the body to fulfill its destiny of converting glucose into energy. And that's the end of the story for that oxygen molecule.

But it's just the beginning of the incredible journey of the newly formed CO_2 molecule. Act Two of this drama is called expiration. As I mentioned above, a byproduct of cellular respiration is carbon dioxide. The same red blood cells — really, the hemoglobin proteins in the red blood cells — that carry O_2 *away* from the lungs also transport CO_2 *back* to the lungs. The migration process works the same way, but in reverse: Blood picks up CO_2 and travels through the bloodstream back to the capillaries that surround the alveoli, across the alveoli wall and back into the tiny air sacs. When the alveoli are full of CO_2, the diaphragm muscle flexes upward, making ribs tighten, and the lungs compress, creating pressure that propels CO_2 up through the bronchioles, bronchi, windpipe, and nose and mouth, back into the atmosphere.

Air Awareness: The average person will cycle through up to 4 million liters of air per year at minimum – more than the capacity of an Olympic swimming pool.[3]

Every inhalation brings in oxygen; every expiration sends out carbon dioxide. This marvel of evolution is called "gas exchange." Every time you breathe, you exchange gas. This function is unique in that it's both involuntary *and* voluntary. Breathing is generally involuntary, like digesting. You don't have to remember to breathe. You don't have to do anything to make it happen. It just does, whether you're awake or asleep. But breathing is also voluntary. You can consciously, right now, take a long, slow, deep breath, hold it for a few seconds, and then exhale at your own pace. Depending on what you're doing, you can mindfully exchange gas faster or slower, deeply or shallowly. Breathing is automatic, yet still something you can adjust.

SHOUT OUT TO THE LUNGS

The liver is a workhorse organ that does so much, producing bile, filtering blood, and storing glucose, to mention just a few of its functions. The gut houses the microbiome, digests food, produces hormones (FYI: It makes more serotonin than the brain does). But pound for pound, the lungs might just be the most fascinating organs in the body.

- **They float**. If removed from the body and thrown in a pool of water, lungs would stay afloat because of the millions of air sacs within.
- **So much blood**. They are reservoirs of it. Five or 6 liters of blood flow through the lungs every minute.[4] They produce blood, too, making ten million platelets per hour.[5]
- **They are *huge*.** The largest internal organ in terms of storage capacity, the lungs hold 500 ml of blood and have the capacity for 6 liters of air. Together, they weigh 2.5 pounds (the heart weighs 8–10 ounces). If you were to lay the bronchi, bronchioles, and alveoli in both lungs end to end, their combined length would be approximately 1,500 miles.
- **They are so efficient**, so big, with so many blood vessels, it takes only seven seconds for an inhaled substance (say, medication or cannabis) to reach the brain.
- **You have two of them**, but unlike other paired organs (e.g., kidneys, ovaries), each lung has a different

structure. The right lung is heavier yet shorter to make room for the liver; it has two bronchi and three lobes. The left lung is lighter and narrower to accommodate the heart; it has one bronchus and two lobes.

- **The lungs can be trained**. Well, not the lungs themselves, but the muscles that surround them. The intercostal muscles of the ribs and the diaphragm can be strengthened with practice to expand lung capacity.

HOW DOES NOT BREATHING KILL YOU?

It is possible for a human being to go double-digit days without sleep. Eventually, your exhausted brain will override willful consciousness by putting you into seconds or minutes of microsleep, even if you aren't aware of it. Rats have died from extreme sleep deprivation, but there is no evidence that people have, at least not directly in a clinical environment.

Due to the incompetence of Austrian prison guards who locked up Andreas Mihavecz and left him in a jail cell, we have proof that a human being can survive eighteen days without food and with very little water. Generally speaking, though, human beings deprived of all water will die in three days.

So how long can you survive without breathing?

In the famous scene in *The Godfather* when Luca Brasi is choked with piano wire in a bar, he goes to sleep with the fishes in twenty-two seconds. Later in the movie, Carlo Rizzi meets a similar fate, garroted in the passenger seat of a car. He fights back and kicks out the windshield as he struggles, but he dies sixteen seconds after airflow to his brain is blocked.

Of course, we don't look to Hollywood for scientific accuracy.

There are many ways to die from asphyxiation, or oxygen

deprivation, that aren't nearly as cinematic as being garroted. The Centers for Disease Control reports that there were nearly 19,000 deaths by asphyxiation in the U.S. in 2018.[6] The causes included drowning, allergic reactions that caused swelling in the upper airways, carbon monoxide poisoning, asthma, choking on food, seizures, opioid overdoses, and strangulation. Spending too much time in environments with only 6 percent O_2 in air (ordinarily, air is 21 percent O_2), such as mines, tunnels, and sewers, can result in CO_2 overdose death.[7] (FYI: The proportion of oxygen in air at high altitudes, such as at the top of Mount Everest, is still 21 percent; the problem is that there is just less air, about one third the amount at sea level.) In these environments, any blockage of the airways puts you at risk for asphyxia, which can lead to brain damage or death.

We know that heart and brain cells start dying rapidly when deprived of oxygen. The brain is greedy for O_2, using 20 percent of the body's supply. And that supply must be *continually* replenished to keep brain cells healthy. But we don't fully understand the mechanisms of what goes on in the brain and heart when air is cut off. Many lab rats have been sacrificed to figure that out. Some research has found that a "brainstorm" of freaked-out neurotransmitters triggers cell death.[8] Acute oxygen deprivation due to pulmonary diseases such as asthma and COPD can trigger a stress response that interferes with cardiac function and can cause a fatal heart attack.[9]

As for the effects of oxygen deprivation, here are common effects:

Within seconds of blocked airflow via suffocation or pressure on the windpipe, a person feels air hunger, that burning sensation in the lungs, a headache, panic, confusion, a sore throat, and blurred vision.

Within one minute, a person sees spots and passes out.

After one minute, brain damage begins.

After five minutes, irreversible brain damage is certain.
After ten minutes, the brain dies.
After fifteen minutes, the rest of the body dies, too.

And yet, despite the wildfire devastation of oxygen deprivation, a human being can survive without taking a breath for 24 minutes and 37 seconds.

This world record for voluntarily holding one's breath goes to Budimir Šobat, a Croatian free diver who, at fifty-six in 2021, floated face down in a swimming pool in Sisak for more than twice as long as a TED Talk about breathing techniques. He did it by practicing and training for three years, and by hyperventilating with 100 percent oxygen from a tank for thirty minutes beforehand.

As stated, normal air is only 21 percent oxygen. Saturating the blood with the pure stuff increases oxygen concentration to such an extent that the ratio of O_2 to CO_2 takes much longer to shift before the lizard brain starts demanding, "Inhale, *now!*" The world record for "static apnea" (holding your breath in water *without* prior hyperventilation with 100 percent oxygen), goes to Branko Petrović, a Serbian free diver who held his breath in a pool in Dubai in 2014 for 11 minutes and 54 seconds.

An ordinary person who hasn't been free diving for years and isn't trained on techniques to control heart rate and to overcome the panicky cues of the respiration drive could not hope to come anywhere near these numbers. The actor Kate Winslet made headlines when she held her breath for over seven minutes while filming an underwater scene in *Avatar: The Way of Water*, with the help of a free diving coach and 100 percent pure oxygen saturation beforehand.

Brava, Kate Winslet. She deserves an Oscar for that alone.

A perplexing question about the domino of breathing: How can you tell if you're doing it well? If you weren't at least proficient, you'd be dead. There are ways to assess if your lungs are reaching their full, incredible potential, which you'll read about next.

TAKEAWAYS

- Breathing is a two-step process of inhaling oxygen and exhaling carbon dioxide, aka "gas exchange." Every breath is filtered by the mucus in your nose, mouth, and airways, to catch pollutants and antigens. Once oxygen reaches the lungs, it's sent into the bloodstream to be delivered all over the body.

- Cellular respiration is the process of turning glucose and O_2 into fuel, creating CO_2 as a byproduct. The whole point of breathing is to create energy so our cells can do what they need to do.

- Air hunger is your breathing drive, the mechanism that forces you to inhale. It's regulated in the brain, too, which constantly monitors the ratio of oxygen to carbon dioxide in your blood.

- The lungs are marvels of evolution that should never be taken for granted.

- Not breathing? It will kill you within minutes. Not advised.

CHAPTER 10

Breathe Assessment Tools

> To prepare to knock down the third Domino
> of Wellness, start by assessing your breathing
> now with these at-home tests.

RESPIRATORY RATE TEST

SHORTNESS OF BREATH TEST

HOLDING BREATH TEST

BLOOD OXYGEN TEST

INHALE-EXHALE DEVICES

CARBON DIOXIDE TOLERANCE TEST

You could go to a pulmonologist and get a full workup of your respiratory capabilities. Or just try these tests at home to get a pretty good idea of how well you take in air.

RESPIRATORY RATE TEST

How many breaths do you take per minute? That number is your respiratory rate. Some smartwatch apps can give you readings of your respiratory rate. Or you can simply count your breaths yourself.

While seated and still, count the number of inhalation-exhalation cycles over sixty seconds. Just breathe normally. Don't take especially deep breaths.

Twelve or fewer cycles indicates excellent overall health.

Thirteen to twenty is normal.

Twenty plus is high and warrants at least a conversation with a medical professional. You might be having a bad allergy day or a panic attack, or have a chronic condition such as asthma or COPD, or an acute case of pneumonia, sepsis, pulmonary embolism, or diabetic ketoacidosis.

My respiratory rate is _____
cycles per minute.

SHORTNESS OF BREATH TEST

Obviously, there is a connection between being physically fit and having strong lungs. Aerobic exercise literally means movement that makes you breathe more deeply and speeds up your heart rate to deliver more oxygen to the muscles and brain. But you don't have to be a marathoner or be able to bench-press 250 pounds to use simple movement to assess the strength of your lungs. What you're measuring here isn't physical fitness, but your lungs' ability to respond to increased oxygen need when you move.

Here's the test.

1. Jog or fast-walk up two flights of stairs.
2. Rate your breathing on a scale of 1 to 4 (ratings below).

A score of 1: You are gasping or panting, sweating, needing two or more minutes to breathe normally again. Perhaps you had to stop between flights to catch your breath or felt pain in your chest. If this is your state, you need to consult a doctor. Dramatic shortness of breath after relatively low exertion is a sign that your brain and other internal organs are not getting enough oxygen.

A score of 2: Your breath is accelerated, and your heart is beating hard. You need over a minute to recover and feeling fatigued from the exertion. You are in okay lung shape. Incorporate more movement and exercise into your day, keep a record, and track improvement.

A score of 3: Your breathing is slightly faster, but it feels good. You need about thirty seconds to recover and are energized by the activity. You are in good lung shape. Deep breathing exercises can get you to a 4.

A score of 4, you were barely fazed by the movement. Your breath is as slow and steady as it was before you jogged up those stairs. You are in excellent lung shape. Congrats!

My shortness of breath score: _____

HOLDING BREATH TEST

1. Sit down (a must; do not hold your breath while standing!)
2. Inhale through your mouth deeply into the belly until you can't take in any more air.
3. Using a stopwatch app, time how long you can hold your breath.

Free divers and movie stars aside, the average adult can hold their breath for thirty to ninety seconds.[1] Anything over a minute is excellent. If you can hold your breath for longer than ninety seconds, as a doctor, I recommend that you pursue a career in synchronized swimming immediately.

The point isn't to make yourself hypoxic (having insufficient oxygen in your blood). It's a test to see if you have healthy, normal lung function. If you can't hold your breath for thirty seconds, it's a sign that you might have a pulmonary condition, a viral infection, anemia, or low air volume capacity. In that case, bring up the issue with your doctor.

Air Awareness Tips: I find it helps not to look at the seconds ticking by. A watched stopwatch moves more slowly. When you feel the respiratory drive kick in, glance at how long you've gone. I find that I get the first sign of discomfort at the thirty-second mark. And then I close my eyes and try to calm down to last for another fifteen or twenty seconds without too much pain or anxiety.

Warning: This isn't an endurance test or a party trick. So don't feel the need to push yourself to the edge of your ability. If you hold your breath for longer than ninety seconds, you might faint.

I can hold my breath for _____ seconds.

BLOOD OXYGEN TEST

In the spring and summer of 2020, during the early days of the COVID-19 pandemic, a device called an electronic pulse oximeter ("pulse ox") started selling out at drug stores and became as common in people's homes as a digital thermometer. A pulse ox device—available for under $20—looks like a miniature sandwich board, with two parts that hinge on one end. The top part has a power button and a digital readout screen. To use it, place your finger between the two parts, release the hinge so your finger rests snugly inside, and then wait about fifteen seconds for two numbers to pop up on the screen. One number measures your SpO_2 percentage or blood oxygen saturation percentage: That is, it measures how much of your red blood cells' hemoglobin is currently bound to oxygen, compared to how much hemoglobin remains unbound. The other number is your BPM (beats per minute), aka heart rate or pulse. Some smartwatches have pulse oximeter apps that are fairly accurate.

An acceptable SpO_2 is 95 to 100 percent. Nearly all your red blood cells are effectively circulating oxygen to tissues and organs that need it.

A reading of 92 to 94 percent is considered low. Not enough oxygen is circulating to tissues and organs. You might have a viral lung infection or some other pulmonary problem. The advice here is to lie down, breathe naturally for a few minutes without holding your breath, and retest. If subsequent readings are below 95, call your doctor and rule out anemia, sleep apnea, asthma, COPD, or pneumonia. Don't wait for the problem to go away on its own.

A reading below 91 means your blood oxygen is dangerously low. Combined with such symptoms as bluish lips, chest pain, a pulse rate of 120 BPM or more, and shortness of breath could mean you are in the midst of a cardiac event. Forget calling the doctor. Go immediately to the emergency room.

INHALE-EXHALE DEVICES

You can buy at-home devices to assess lung capacity and airflow strength. Usually, such gizmos are for people with pulmonary illnesses such as asthma, emphysema, or chronic bronchitis. But they are gaining in popularity for use among athletes looking to improve those metrics. They're relatively inexpensive and worth checking out if you're curious about your lung functionality and/or want to train and strengthen your diaphragm and intercostal muscles.

The two main options:

A peak flow meter. This handheld tool measures airflow rate by testing how fast you can blast air out of your lungs into a mouthpiece.

A spirometer. Another handheld device, a spirometer measures exhale force (like the peak flow meter), as well as lung volume capacity during inhales.

Those who prefer a high-tech approach can check out gizmos like the Airofit Pro "breathing trainer" device that you put in your mouth and exhale for measurements of respiratory rate, lung capacity, and other data. Prices range from $129 to $349 for the latest version. Similar electronic devices, some with smartphone links, are available online for over $100.

A low-tech rudimentary plastic tube device tests both exhale power and inhale volume. I bought one online for $20. It's as basic as they come. It has three tubes, each with a plastic ball inside. The tubes connect to a mouthpiece. To measure lung capacity, you put the mouthpiece between your lips and then inhale steadily through the mouth for as long as you can. The suction creates a vacuum effect that lifts the plastic balls inside their tubes. If you can keep those balls elevated for a count of three to five, you have excellent lung capacity. Turning the device upside down, you can measure airflow strength by placing the mouthpiece between your lips and exhaling steadily until the lungs are completely empty, keeping those balls elevated within the tubes for a count of three to five.

If you try an at-home device and find that your peak flow is weak, don't freak out. Now you know that you have something to work on and room for improvement. I love a project, and what better one than strengthening your airflow?

CARBON DIOXIDE TOLERANCE TEST

This test was designed by Brian Mackenzie, a human performance specialist, founder of Shift Health, and cofounder and president of the Health and Human Performance Foundation, as a way to measure "how sensitive we are to CO_2, where our nervous system is, and how reactive we are to stress."[2]

1. Sit or lie down for a few minutes, breathing normally.
2. Take three normal nose-only inhalation-exhalation cycles.
3. Take one big, full nasal inhale.
4. At the peak of that breath, start a stopwatch and begin slowly, steadily exhaling until you have nothing left to exhale.

My carbon dioxide tolerance test time is _____ seconds.

If you exhaled for under 30 seconds, per Mackenzie, you are probably highly stressed, are not an athlete and don't exercise daily, and/or are recovering from an illness.

If you exhaled for 30 to 45, you are still stressed, exercise sporadically, and have room for improvement in your overall health.

If you exhaled for 45 to 60 seconds, you are active, with a balanced nervous system, and probably already have a breathing practice and exercise routine.

If you exhaled for over 60 seconds, you are a fine physical specimen, possibly a professional or competitive athlete and probably a freak of nature (my words, not Mackenzie's).

Doing any one of these tests provides some idea of your respiratory health. But taken as a whole, you will undoubtedly notice some patterns. Don't be discouraged if your scores aren't what you thought they could be. Accept it and move on to the next chapter, where you will find out why your breathing isn't as optimal as you'd like it to be. We'll improve on that when you enact the Sleep-Drink-Breathe Plan, but you have to undo bad habits before you establish new ones.

TAKEAWAYS

- Check your respiratory rate—how many times you inhale and exhale per minute when at rest—for a great baseline assessment of your breathing. For an adult, less than twenty is considered normal. For a yogi, less than twelve. More than twenty-five, you could have a medical condition or be in the middle of a panic attack.
- Breath-holding time of up to ninety seconds indicates healthy lungs. Less than thirty seconds means you might have restricted breathing due to illness or age.

- Jog up two flights of stairs as a shortness of breath test, to get an idea of your lung fitness level. If you gasp and pant, you have some breathwork to do.
- Airflow strength testers are most commonly used by people with pulmonary illnesses, but anyone curious about their breathing health can get one to assess their peak flow. Prices vary, depending on how high-tech the device is.

CHAPTER 11

Troubleshooting Breathe

Inhale and exhale. We do it constantly and have since the moment we were born. Despite all that experience, many of us have bad breathing habits.

THE CONSEQUENCES

poor cognitive performance
stress and inflammation
heart problems
sleep issues
compromised immunity

THE TOP SIX BAD BREATHING HABITS

taking it for granted
too shallow
too high
too fast
too mouthy
holding it

In my initial research into breathing and various techniques that can improve pulmonary and general health, I spoke to several people about how they felt about their own breathing skills. Nearly all of them said things like "I don't need to work on my breathing technique. I've been breathing my entire life with no problem, so I must be doing it right!"

True. If you weren't breathing, you would not be alive to question whether you're doing it well. However, just because you are doing something does not mean you are doing it to the best of your ability, or even using it in a way that could provide even greater benefit.

A crucial Domino of Wellness, breathing is often overlooked as a tweakable biobehavior. The general public might be aware that taking a deep breath makes you feel less stressed out. That's what Grandma always said (and she was right). But did Grandma, or doctors, or the media, explain why or how breathing can calm us down? Nope.

Everyone knows the conventional (and not entirely accurate) benchmarks about sleep and hydration. Ask anyone, and they'll probably say, "You need eight hours of sleep per night" and "You should drink eight glasses of water per day." Some of the consequences for insufficient sleep and inadequate hydration exist in the public consciousness. Again, ask anyone, and they'll probably say, "Not sleeping makes you feel groggy, exhausted, and cranky" or "Not drinking enough causes dehydration."

But breathing benchmarks — like a recommended daily allowance (which we have for vitamins and minerals) for air — and consequences for breathing suboptimally are not common knowledge. Practically no one is going to say with a straight face, "Shoot for 15,000 slow belly breaths per day." But that is a realistic and helpful goal! The alternative, just breathing the way you always have, might not be serving you. There *are* mental, emotional, and physical consequences to the same-old breathing style.

Poor cognitive performance. Memory, concentration, atten-tion, decision-making, and problem solving are all aspects of cogni-tive function, or mental sharpness. For their 2021 study, researchers in Korea set out to find a link between a particular inefficient breath-ing habit ("oral breathing") and cognitive function. They hooked up twenty-two healthy young men to a functional MRI (fMRI) machine and asked them to do memory tests while breathing through their nose or mouth. While nose breathing, the subjects' brain regions for memory were significantly more activated and connected than the mouth breathers'.[1]

> *Air Awareness*: Oral breathing impairs cognitive function and is a disadvantage for any intellectual pursuit. Your nose knows!

I'll explain nose vs. mouth breathing in depth in a bit, but the takeaway here is that how you breathe makes a real difference in how you think.

Stress and inflammation. Way back in the Sleep chapters, I talked about the circadian rhythm of the stress hormone cortisol. In the Drink chapters, I explained how free radicals cause oxidative stress, which leads to chronic inflammation. Well, there's another aspect of stress and inflammation that really comes into play with breathing.

You have two nervous systems in the body: the sympathetic (the fight-flight-freeze stress response) and the parasympathetic (the rest-digest-socialize-calm response). Only one of these systems is "on" at any given time. Although your mind might think you can be both emotionally aroused and relaxed concurrently, your body is not as subtle. According to your nervous system, you are either stressed or calm, never both.

A big problem in our society is chronic stress due to the constant demands and pressures of modern life. For too many of us, stress is our default setting, and we are so used to it that we don't even realize we're in this state. But your body always knows, because your sympathetic nervous system is working overtime, locked in the "on" position. In fight-flight-freeze, the adrenal glands dump cortisol into the system, which speeds up the heart, raises blood pressure, and inhibits digestion and other functions. Cortisol-overload hormonal imbalance is a known cause of inflammation,[2] the red-hot and puffy internal environment that is associated with conditions such as heart disease, metabolic syndrome, arthritis, and stroke.

Stress → inflammation → disease

The sympathetic nervous system switches "on" in response to psychological or physical cues. A psychological cue is when you feel under threat. It could be due to a harsh email from a coworker, traffic, a scary scene in a movie, an actual violent attack. A physical cue that triggers the stress response is rapid breathing or panting. You don't even have to feel scared for the body to think it's under attack. If you pant, the adrenal glands believe you need blood redirected to your muscles and heart so you can fight or flee, so they release cortisol.

Rapid breathing → stress → inflammation → disease

Heart issues. The heart and left lung cozy up next to each other. Both lungs are, essentially, filled with blood, laced throughout with capillaries. The cardiovascular and respiratory systems work closely together to carry oxygen from the lungs to organs and tissues, and tote carbon dioxide from organs and tissues back to the lungs to be expelled from the body. These two systems are connected. The phrase used in science is "cardiorespiratory coupling." Breathing improperly — too fast, too slow, too shallow — negatively affects the heart. We're talking about diminished aortic function, higher blood pressure, elevated heart rate.[3]

Sleep issues. Sleep apnea is a category of sleep disorder that is literally about faulty breathing. But improper breathing habits can cause insomnia as well. Rapid breath cycles can trigger the fight-or-flight response as well as symptoms like high blood pressure and heart rate. Those physiological conditions would be ideal if you were being chased through Tokyo by Godzilla. But when you lie down in bed at the end of a stressful, exhausting day, fast, shallow breathing puts your body into an overexcited state that is the opposite of the quiet calm you need to drift off. And when you don't drift off, anxiety can escalate. More cortisol, less likelihood of falling asleep. The vicious cycle all started with improper breathing style.

Compromised immunity. The cardiovascular system's arteries, veins, and capillaries circulate blood throughout the body to bring nutrients and oxygen to every cell, tissue, and organ. It's powered by a pump, the heart itself. Running alongside the cardiovascular system is the lymphatic system. It circulates lymphatic fluid and acts as the body's sewer. It collects cellular waste, bacteria, inflammatory chemicals, and toxins, filters them, and sends them to the kidneys for elimination. The lymphatic system does not have a pump to keep fluid moving. Its circulation depends on valves in the vessels and our moving around.

You need lymphatic fluid to move at a healthy speed, with enough pressure to push through the body's filters, including 600 to 800 lymph nodes. Not enough pressure, those nodules get clogged. If that happens, toxins pile up inside your body like trash on the street during a garbage strike.

What does all this have to do with breathing? About half of your lymph nodes are in the abdomen. When you flex the diaphragm, the nodes in the area get squeezed and wrung out, unclogging debris. Deep abdominal breathing also stimulates lymph flow and speeds things up inside vessels. Free-flowing fluids means more pressure to push through the filters, keeping them clear and preventing toxin pileup. The diaphragm is like the lymphatic system's manual pump. To make it work, you have to crank it yourself.

If you breathe into the chest, as opposed to the abdomen, lymphatic pressure drops. Nodes swell. Toxic sludge and germs stay in the body instead of getting filtered and dumped. That leads to increased inflammation, cell degeneration, and susceptibility to illness.

But there's even more to the breathing-immunity connection. Along with filtering waste, the lymphatic system produces lymphocytes, which are a kind of white blood cell, immunity frontline defenders that attack and kill bacteria, fungi, parasites, and viruses. If the lymphatic fluid isn't flowing, those white blood cells can't get where they're needed to go to fight invaders, and you wind up getting more infections and sicknesses.

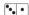

Even more consequences are specific to certain styles of suboptimal inhaling and exhaling, as I'll explain as I go through the Top Six Bad Breathing Habits that you might not even realize you're doing. Air Awareness is the first step! So take a deep breath and then read on.

BAD BREATHING HABIT #1: TAKING IT FOR GRANTED

Just because you can do a thing doesn't mean you're doing it to the best of your ability. There is always potential for improvement, whether you're riding a bike, writing a book, or inhaling O_2 and exhaling CO_2. Breathing is one of the most crucial bodily functions you've got. It converts sugar into energy. It can quiet anxiety and reduce stress. It supports the immune system. It delivers nutrients to hungry cells and takes out the body's trash. Knowing all of that, why wouldn't you make an effort to boost your breathing skills? I'm not asking you to make major changes. Small tweaks will bring big rewards, especially as you get older.

Your lungs are in their prime at age twenty-five, when they are fully developed. By the time you hit thirty-five, they begin their slow crawl to degradation. By eighty, "pulmonary function and aerobic capacity each decline by [as much as] 40 percent," according to a 2016 report in the *European Respiration Journal.*[4] Age-associated diminishment of lung capacity isn't just for smokers and non-exercises. It happens to *everyone.*

Some of the changes that are in store for your respiratory system[5]:

As **alveoli** age, they go from perky grapes on the vine to saggy, dried-up raisins you find in the back of the pantry.

The **diaphragm** weakens over time, so you can't take in as much air or exhale as much with each breath.

Ribs that stretch to allow your lungs to fill up become brittle and less elastic with age. People over fifty: If you've noticed that climbing stairs gets harder each year, you can blame your bones.

Mucosal tissue in the respiratory system diminishes with age, making its germ-catching properties less effective. During the pandemic, seniors were far more likely than younger people to have serious COVID-19 symptoms and to die of it. Their weakened respiratory mucus contributed to that grim statistic. What's more, the brain signal that says "Cough now" gets quieter over time, so seniors aren't hacking up germs and excess mucus that clogs airways. They wind up getting sick and having reduced oxygen intake.

It's hard to imagine that one day, something you have always done with ease will be compromised through no fault of your own. As my eighty-five-year-old friend puts it, "Aging is not for the young. It's way too scary."

But you can strengthen your respiratory system at any time to slow the aging process and keep your lungs in good shape throughout your life. The first minor adjustment to make is to flip the mental switch and stop thinking of breathing as the body's job. Instead, think of it as a superpower you can master and a skill you can use to improve your health and wellness and to change your mind and body for the better every single day.

BAD BREATHING HABIT #2: TOO SHALLOW

We draw life-sustaining oxygen into our lungs to be distributed via the bloodstream throughout the body. That single, crucial objective is compromised by shallow breaths.

Taking in little puffs of air, mostly through the mouth, using the ribs' intercostal muscles is a pattern called "thoracic breathing." (The thorax is the area of the body between the neck and the abdomen, aka the chest.)

There are some understandable reasons to take shallow breaths into the chest, as opposed to deep ones into the abdomen. For instance, asthma sufferers and pneumonia patients might be incapable of drawing air deep into the belly. If you broke a rib or just had an appendectomy and it's physically painful to expand the diaphragm, by all means, breathe into the chest.

Along with reduced oxygen intake, shallow breathing has been associated with anxiety attacks. Per a 2019 study, people tend to breathe through the mouth and into the chest in times of emotional stress and anxiety.[6] So if you are, say, in the throes of a panic attack, your body shifts into a fight-flight-freeze sympathetic nervous response with the accompanying cortisol, increased heart rate, and shallow breathing. Some studies have found that shallow breathing can actually *cause* a panic attack. For a 2017 study published in *Science*, researchers at Stanford University located a subpopulation of neurons in the breathing pacemaker part of the brain, the locus coeruleus, that signals the brain's arousal center (not sexual arousal—any kind of arousal, including stress). The scientists removed those neurons in mice, effectively cutting the lines of communication between breathing speed and stress. Next, they put the mice into a panic-inducing situation that would, in normal mice, make them start to breathe shallowly and rapidly. But the brain-altered mice continued breathing normally and acted completely calm. The conclusion of this experiment? By controlling breathing depth and speed, you can influence "higher-order brain function."[7]

Long-term shallow breathing has been associated with low levels of lymphocytes, the immunity foot soldiers that fight germs.[8]

Still think breathing style isn't that big a deal?

Air Awareness: Your breath will control you unless you learn to control it. If your current breathing style is to inhale little puffs into the chest, you take in less oxygen, clog the lymphatic system, and make fewer immunity soldiers. You could also exacerbate a panic attack in progress or trigger a new one.

LEAVE NO LOBES BEHIND

You have five lobes in your two lungs: the upper, middle, and lower lobes in the right lung and upper and lower lobes in the left lung. During my morning routine of taking fifteen deep breaths, I visualize each lobe filling up with each breath. First, I inhale deep into the bottom lobes, flexing the diaphragm. Then I take another quick inhale that expands the ribs and fills the middle and top lobes. Another technique is to alternate between chest and abdominal breathing to fill every nook and cranny of both lungs with air. It feels amazing. Instantly invigorating.

BAD BREATHING HABIT #3: TOO HIGH

Quick exercise: Take a breath. Do your shoulders rise? When you exhale, do they fall? If so, you are "vertical breathing" into the upper lobes and leaving the middle and lower lobes high and dry. You're not taking in as much oxygen as you could, and you are potentially allowing excessive mucus to build up in the lower lobes.

By breathing vertically, you rely on upper body muscles, like those in your chest, shoulders, back, and neck. Overuse of those muscle groups can cause stiffness and aches. Habitual vertical breathers often contend with chronic back or neck pain.[9] It's a chicken-egg situation. If you have back pain, you might compensate by slumping or slouching. In that posture, it's harder to take a deep breath, so you wind up taking vertical breaths instead, which make you tense your neck, back, and shoulder muscles. You can easily see how the cycle of back pain, bad posture, and high breathing reinforces itself.

Whenever I see someone rubbing their neck or shoulders, my first thought is, "They need to breathe horizontally." No matter how many massages you get or Epsom salt baths your take, if you breathe vertically, your upper body muscles are going to be overworked.

The alternative is "horizontal breathing," when the breathing motion expands the abdomen outward. The belly rounds as if a baby alien were about to pop out. Horizonal breathing is the ideal way to take in more air, send oxygen quickly into the bloodstream, squeeze lymph nodes, and torque up maximal lymphatic pressure.

BAD BREATHING HABIT #4: TOO FAST

Back in Chapter 10, I asked you to assess your respiratory rate or the number of inhalation-exhalation cycles per minute while breathing normally.

In a healthy body, a person's at-rest breathing rate is twelve to twenty breaths per minute at medium depth, bringing in several liters at a time. Healthy people ordinarily inhale for one or two seconds, and exhale for two or three, so a typical cycle lasts for three to five seconds.

Having these numbers and an awareness about the speed of your breathing can help you mindfully slow things down. Fast breathing isn't really a choice; it's either a sign of respiratory limitation or a habit. But breathing problems can be treated, and habits can be broken. Speed of breathing is a key area you can train yourself to improve and reap the benefit of emotional regulation and stress reduction.

For an adult, a respiratory rate over twenty indicates that you might be hyperventilating. The cause might be excessive exercise, anger, or a panic attack. Even an intense sob fest could make you overbreathe. The issue isn't necessarily the speed of your breaths but that you're taking in only a thimbleful of air when you need liters by volume. The hyperventilation pattern is too little oxygen in and too much carbon dioxide out, which can throw you into a state of hypoxia (lack of oxygen) that might lead to dizziness, confusion, muscle cramps and spasms, chest pains, and fainting.

A respiratory rate of over twenty-eight is a major red flag, and a very good reason to seek medical attention immediately. If you're just sitting on the couch and breathing so fast you can barely catch your breath, it could mean you have a respiratory illness like COPD, asthma, pneumonia, or a pulmonary embolism, or that you're in the midst of a heart attack, a drug overdose, or an intense pain experience.

RESPIRATORY RATES BY AGE

Do not panic if your baby seems to be breathing very rapidly! It's normal for newborns to inhale and exhale as fast as a cat. Here are some rates for people of all ages:

- Newborns (up to six weeks): 30–40 breaths per minute
- Babies (six weeks–one year): 25–40
- Toddlers (one–three years): 20–30
- Children (three–ten years): 17–23
- Teens (ten–eighteen years): 15–18
- Young Adults: 12–20
- Middle-aged Adults: 18–25
- Young Seniors: 12–28
- Over Eighty: 10–30[10]

Air Awareness: As a rule, the mouth is for eating; the nose is for breathing.

BAD BREATHING HABIT #5:
TOO MOUTHY

We have evolved to be able to breathe through both the nose and mouth. If one part is unavailable, we have the other to keep us alive. So if you have terrible congestion from a cold, you can still take in air by the mouth. If your mouth is eating, kissing, talking, or whatever else a mouth does, you have two nostrils at your disposal.

Why is the mouth the inferior choice for breathing?

Calling someone a "mouth breather" is not a compliment. The Urban Dictionary's definition of *mouthbreather* is "someone who is really dumb." Of course, inhaling through the mouth has nothing to do with intelligence. People who have been doing so since childhood most likely have severe allergies, narrow nostril pathways, a structural oral problem, a deviated septum, or a cartilage deformity.[11] Children who suck their thumbs often press on the palate of the mouth, which decreases the size of nasal cavities, making it harder for them to get enough air by nose breathing. If a child's blockage or thumb sucking is never addressed, they can fall into the habit of mouth breathing. Unfortunately, as they grow up, they can develop "mouth breather face," characterized by a receding chin, a long, narrow face, droopy eyes, large forehead, flat nose, and a head that juts forward over the shoulders. It's not a great look and does make a less than intelligent impression.

Adults who mouth breathe do it out of habit, or they're dealing with allergies, congestion, sleep apnea,[12] or swollen tonsils or adenoids that partially block airways. Mouth breathing during sleep is common and can indicate an obstructive disorder. Unless you have a helpful partner who kicks you in bed when you snore, the only way to know if you sleep with your mouth open is waking up with classic symptoms: dry mouth, cracked lips, scratchy throat, and brain fog.

The biggest danger of sleeping with your mouth open isn't bad breath, oral yeast infection, gum disease, or cavities (although these are potential outcomes). It's, metaphorically, letting the flies in. Every floating germ, dust mite, or environmental toxin has a golden invitation to enter your mouth and throat. Because mouth breathing dries and irritates your throat, it might have microtears, the ideal home for bacteria and viruses to nestle into. During the pandemic, scientists did a ton of research about transmission. One 2021 study found that mouth breathers were more likely to be infected and to transmit the virus.[13] Basically, breathing through your mouth is like putting leaded gas in your car.

OSA: A SLEEP-BREATHE TRAIN WRECK

Hyperventilating by day just might do a 180 and turn into *hypo*-ventilating by night. Overbreathing becomes underbreathing—or no breathing—if you have obstructive sleep apnea. If you have OSA, gas exchange slows down to such a degree that the brain becomes deprived of oxygen. Those with OSA wake up multiple times per night just to breathe. The wake-ups might be so brief that sufferers don't even know they're happening. Undiagnosed OSA sufferers are constantly exhausted from poor-quality rest.

If you suspect you have OSA, go to an ENT or a sleep doctor to confirm it. Classic symptoms are snoring, irritability, difficulty concentrating, feeling tired despite spending hours "asleep." Take this seriously! The risks of lack of oxygen during sleep are life-threatening; they include heart disease, stroke, dementia, and death.

Air Awareness Alert: If you think that you can't die from sleep apnea, I am unfortunately here to tell you that it's very possible. One of my best friends and patients (this book is partially dedicated to him) had this happen. He had some level of compromised lung function, as he was quite big, he had significant sleep apnea, and we had him on a great CPAP, losing weight, and really moving in the right direction. As former law enforcement, he knew how to be disciplined and really focused. He lost 80 pounds, was working out daily, and was significantly happier. But over time, his habits started to revert. He gained some weight and had to have his CPAP increased, and then it became less comfortable. He may have had some artery blockage, and when you lie on your back with 275 pounds of body weight, it's tough to have the energy to breathe, so your oxygen levels can get depressed. Over a night, this can turn into a critical situation, especially when you remove your CPAP due to discomfort, which he did. One night his apnea resulted in a severe cardiac arrest, and he could not be saved. He was one of my best friends, and I miss him dearly, almost every day. If you decide NOT to do anything about your breathing for yourself, I want to remind everyone that you should never underestimate the effect of your presence in others' lives.

BAD BREATHING HABIT #6: HOLDING IT

Someone must have told you at some point during your life, "Don't forget to breathe."

Unintentional breath holding happens when people are nervous or they are anticipating bad news or scary feelings. The last time I found myself holding my breath, I was about to open an email from my doctor with test results I'd been waiting for. It's common for people to hold their breath in high-pressure situations such as meetings or during exams.

It's also happened to me when I've been concentrating very hard while writing (this book). The phrases "email apnea" and "screen apnea" were originally coined by writer and former Apple and Microsoft executive Linda Stone. As she writes in her blog,[14] the terms refer to the "temporary cessation of breath or shallow breathing while working (or playing!) in front of screens." For her own research, she invited 200 people over and studied their respiratory rate and heart rate variability while they worked on screens to see if they held their breath. Eighty percent did. The 20 percent who didn't were athletes, dancers, musicians—people who'd been trained in breathwork before.

Whether anxious or focused, people tend to clench their muscles, including the respiratory ones. Imagine walking down a dark street and suddenly hearing a suspicious noise. The first thing you'd do is freeze and stop breathing. It's a natural reflex, like a cat freezing in place right before it pounces on prey or a toy. That pause, a built-in part of the stress response, gives you a second to decide what it's going to be — fight or flight.

What's more, in a focus- or anxiety-related clamped-down state, breathing is just physiologically harder. The conscious brain might be furiously active, but the diaphragm is temporarily immobile. Just a few seconds of not breathing is enough to throw off the O_2 to CO_2 ratio, and suddenly the body freaks out because it's not getting enough oxygen. Cue the sympathetic nervous system response and cortisol dump.

We are on screens for hours and hours per day. We receive untold emails and texts, and each one — in particular, unexpected and anxiety-producing ones — can trigger a breath-holding pattern. If that pattern turns into an unintentional habit that you might not even be aware of, you can wind up living, continually, in stress mode, inflamed, at risk for burnout, and exhausted.

Air Awareness: You know what really helps with unintentional breath holding? Getting up and moving around. Being sedentary is a circulation issue, and anything that affects the cardiovascular system affects the pulmonary system. Those systems are the cutest couple, and they have such a mutually beneficial relationship. What's good for one is good for the other. A sedentary life is a major risk factor for poor circulation because the heart, a muscle, weakens with disuse. Aerobic exercise – the kind that makes you breathe harder – increases blood flow and therefore gas exchange.

Next up, all the ways you can tweak breathing for wild benefits that, I promise, have never occurred to you before. There is so much good in taking a long, slow, deep breath. And I can't wait to tell you about it.

TAKEAWAYS

- Let's make air awareness as standard a health goal as getting good sleep and sufficient hydration. Like those other Dominos of Wellness, breathing well can positively affect your health profoundly.
- Poor breathing habits — too shallow, too high, too fast, bad posture — trigger the stress response. Chronic stress causes inflammation, which can cause horrible diseases. Besides that, bad breathing habits lower immunity, make you susceptible to viruses and germs, and bring about neck, shoulder, and back pain.
- Mouth breathing, don't get me started. It's a mess. It opens the barn door to viral and bacterial infections, causes dental issues, is dehydrating — and it's just a less efficient way to draw air into the lungs.
- Accidentally holding your breath, which happens when you concentrate hard or are scared or surprised instantly, sends you into fight-or-flight mode and triggers a cortisol release. Too much cortisol causes hormonal imbalance. We're aiming for whole-body balance (homeostasis), which means regulating the stress response, not triggering it.

CHAPTER 12

Breathe for the Win

> *Breathe in health and wellness. Breathe out stress and anxiety. Inhale new techniques that help you control your emotions. Exhale bad habits that are harming your immunity.*

BREATHE DOMINO GOODIES

weight loss

reduced stress and inflammation

more energy

mental clarity

pain reduction

longer life

hot sex

TOP SIX CHANGES TO BREATHE IN

Use your nose.

Strengthen the diaphragm.

Stand (and sit) tall.

Clear phlegm.

Master the techniques.

Get blood moving.

Saving the best for last. Of the three Dominos of Wellness, tweaking your breathing might be the easiest to do. You don't need a bed to sleep in or a stainless steel water bottle to drink out of. All that's required of you is a little bit of commitment and the willingness to do something you already do in a slightly different way. The rewards for this minimal effort are so worth it! What you stand to gain if you breathe in change:

Weight loss. Remarkable research has found a connection between doing a breathing practice and a lower BMI.[1] A recent Indian study looked at yogic breathing (Bhramari pranayama and OM chanting) and the effect on lung function of their eighty-two healthy adult participants. The intervention group practiced the breathing techniques for ten minutes a day, six days a week for two weeks. Not only did they make huge improvements on their peak flow (exhale force) and other pulmonary factors, but they enjoyed *significant weight reductions*, too, just from daily chanting and breathing.

How does that work? It's possible certain **breathing practices reduce hunger**.[2] For a 2017 study, American and Ukrainian researchers divided their sixty subjects into an intervention group that did Qigong exercises on an empty stomach; another group did deep breathing exercises instead. To get accurate info about the participants' subjective sense of hunger, the scientists checked their stomach pH and intestinal pressure measurements in addition to self-reported assessments. The group that did the Qigong breathing technique had an increase in stomach pH, meaning it got more alkaline, possibly due to a reduction of gastric acid. And their intestinal pressure decreased, so they felt less urgency to eat. The researchers concluded that doing the specific technique between meals or while fasting is a viable technique to control hunger. (For specific details, go to page 225.)

Science has also found that a breathing practice **increases metabolic rate**. For a 2018 Korean study, researchers took two measurements of their thirty-eight subjects before and after they did a diaphragm breathing exercise: maximal oxygen uptake (how much they could draw in) and resting metabolic rate (how much energy they burned just by being alive). A short series of deep belly breathing improved their O_2 intake and sped up metabolic rate.[3] By just sitting and sucking air into your belly, you can stoke fat burn.

One last weight-loss factor: **Breathing increases leptin release**. Leptin is the satiety hormone. When you've had enough hummus wrap, leptin secretions signal to your brain, "Don't eat another bite." Without this hormone, people might never know when to put down the fork. In a recent study, scientist split a group of sixty-eight overweight and obese people into a ninety-minute per day walk group and a ninety-minute per day yoga group. Both groups got the same healthy diet. Although all participants decreased BMI and waist and hip measurements and gained more lean mass, only the yoga group — deep breathing being a part of that practice — increased leptin blood levels.[4] Leptin isn't the most reliable signal for people with a long history of dieting and binging. If hunger and satiety hormonal messages are repeatedly ignored by the conscious mind, you stop hearing them. If years of dieting have made your satiety signals too quiet to hear, exercise plus deep breathing turns up the volume, making "I'm full" messages harder to ignore.

Air Awareness: For those at risk of Alzheimer's disease: A 2023 study found that doing a slow breathing practice for twenty to forty minutes per day stimulates the vagus nerve pathway, which clears dementia-related proteins amyloid beta and tau in the brain.[5]

Reduced stress and inflammation. Apologies if you are sick of hearing me say that stress causes oxidative stress, which turns into inflammation, and that chronic inflammation is going to kill us all.

I'm sick of saying it! But you can't ignore it. As individuals and as a society, we have to learn how to manage stress and anxiety to prevent epidemic levels of stress- and inflammation-related conditions, including burnout, heart disease, stroke, autoimmune disease, diabetes, arthritis, COPD, dementia,[6] and mood disorders.

Since you can breathe yourself out of fight-or-flight mode, you can practically reduce inflammation at will. I could present a thousand studies on this. The overwhelming findings are that diaphragmatic breathing (slow, into the belly) lowers heart rate.[7] It drops cortisol levels.[8] It tones the vagus nerve, the body's all-important "wanderer" nerve that, when stimulated by deep breathing, switches off fight-or-flight and switches on the rest-and-digest parasympathetic nervous system.[9] Breathing improves your ability to regulate emotions, which is a lot better and healthier than feeling that you are at the mercy of your moods and feelings.

More energy. In Sanskrit, *prana* means breath, and it also means energy. According to the ancient Indians who invented yoga, breathing is the fire that fuels the body. (In a purely biological sense, that is true; as you recall, oxygen "burns" glucose into energy.) Depending on the technique you use, breathing has the potential to give you a quick burst of energy (get-up-and-go) and alertness (mental vigor). By taking long, deep, rhythmic breaths, you enhance oxygen concentration and blood circulation, rocketing nutrients into your muscles and brain. An O_2 boost is like a tiny cocaine jolt, minus the tooth grinding and brain rot.

I talk a lot about the two autonomic nervous systems—the sympathetic (high alert) and the parasympathetic (at ease). Fast breathing or panting activates high-alert mode, a cortisol release, elevated heart rate and blood pressure, and the increased flow of oxygen and blood to the extremities so you can run away from the tiger (real, imagined, or metaphorical) that's chasing you. A chronic state of stress causes major problems, such as oxidative stress and inflammation, but an acute stress response might be just the energy hit you need to power through a difficult task during a trying day. You can "game" your nervous systems to access quick energy via sharp inhalations in rapid succession, and then, when you need to calm down, you can use a different technique to switch off fight-or-flight and go into rest-and-digest.

When you learn to turn on and off the stress response with breath, you gain energy from that mastery. You're no longer sapped by feeling out of control of your emotions or bogged down by negative ones. By breathing away muscle tension, you use less energy and can redirect energy toward doing more fun and productive things.

Mental clarity. As for mental benefits, deep breathing increases blood oxygen saturation and circulation, so more O_2 reaches the brain faster. That's good for cognition, the ability to focus, solve problems, make decisions, be creative. In a 2017 Chinese study, scientists had half of their forty participants do twenty intensive breathing training sessions over eight weeks; the control group didn't change their routine at all. Both groups were tested before and after the study for attention span, negative affect (bad mood), and cortisol levels in their saliva. The deep breathing group showed significant improvements in sustained attention, positive affect, and stress compared to their own pre-study levels and the control group.[10]

Air Awareness for menopausal women: Having hot flashes, night sweats, irritability, and mood swings? Studies show that if you spend fifteen minutes a day slowing your breathing rate of fifteen to twenty cycles per minute down to five or seven, you can abate hot flashes in the moment and prevent future ones.[11] Hopefully, calming breath can also help you not want to kill random strangers at Trader Joe's.

Pain reduction. Slow breathing techniques have been proven to reduce the intensity and agony of pain for people who suffer from chronic conditions such as fibromyalgia,[12] lower back pain,[13] and headache, per the American Migraine Foundation.[14] The question is, how can doing something as simple as breathing lower one's perception of pain? German scientists figured that out by subjecting sixteen healthy adults to hot and cold stimuli while having them do deep, slow breathing techniques. By tracking the subjects' pain experience via sympathetic nervous system response, researchers noted decreased stress from pain and better mood in the subjects while they were doing the breathing techniques.[15] Pain is pain; it exists or it doesn't. But by adding breathing to the equation, you can mitigate your reaction to unpleasant sensations so they don't bother you as much.

Longer life. We live long by preventing deadly disease and being able to recover from illness. Well, stronger immunity[16] and lowered blood pressure[17] have been associated with a deep breathing practice. It can improve pulmonary function, even in elderly smokers whose lifestyle choices would ordinarily shorten their lifespan.[18] There is evidence that breathing exercises as part of a regimen of mindfulness-based recovery practices can lengthen telomeres—the endcaps of DNA that erode over time, signaling a decrease in longevity—among breast cancer survivors.[19] Breathe in wellness; breathe out illness. It really is as simple, and beautiful, as that.

OXYGEN STARTS WITH O

Typically, leading up to orgasm, there's a lot of shallow, rapid breathing, possibly panting. Right before orgasm, it's quite common for people to hold their breath in what I'll call "sex apnea."

When you are in the throes, you're probably not thinking about breathing. But if you can tear your attention away from the task at hand and turn your focus to breathing for just a moment, you can double your pleasure.

Any kind of arousal—whether responding to sex, stage fright, being chased by a tiger—involves the same physiological response: cortisol dump and increased heart rate, breathing rate, and blood pressure, as well as a rush of blood to the muscles (so you can run away!). But what you *really* want during sexual arousal is increased blood and oxygen flow to the sex organs. Without it, erections of the penis and clitoris are weak or nonexistent. When you hold your breath on the verge of orgasm, the body reacts by redirecting O_2-rich blood away from your core and into the extremities, the opposite direction you want it to go.

So tune into your breathing pattern during sex, and if you do hold your breath on the verge of orgasm, break that habit and make a new one. Intentionally inhale deeply through the nose into the belly, as low as you can go, and exhale through the mouth in a controlled pace. Visualize the air reaching your genitals and flooding them to Big O_2 Energy.

Practice while alone to get used to doing this. At first, doing the technique might distract you and knock you off the path. But once you get a hang of it, you'll love practicing it again and again, alone or with a partner. You will find that breathing during orgasm makes it last longer and feel more intense, and it brings on super powerful contractions.

Finally, it's time to learn specific techniques to inhale health, smarts, and happiness and exhale stress, fogginess, and fatigue. Here are the Top Six Changes to Breathe In:

BREATHE CHANGE #1:
USE YOUR NOSE

You were designed to breathe primarily through the nose. It's just a more effective and efficient way to take in oxygen and expel carbon dioxide. It also warms air as it's coming in, which your lungs appreciate.

Since the nasal cavity is narrower than the oral cavity, inhaling through your nostrils creates 50 percent more resistance, which has a wind tunnel effect inside your sinuses. The airflow is pressurized as it rockets into your windpipe, resulting in an increase of up to 20 percent in oxygen intake.[20] And because of the smaller exit ramp, nose breathing extends the length of exhales, which has the benefit of keeping you in parasympathetic calm mode.

Nostril hairs might not be the most attractive part of the nasal apparatus. But they do a great job of filtering bacteria, dust, and other harmful substances you might inhale. Your other airways have cilia, little hair-like protrusions, that trap pathogens, too. But nose hairs are your first, best defense against them. Trim them at your own risk. The mucus that lines your nasal cavities keeps the area moist and traps bugs and debris incredibly well. If you breathe through your mouth, much more gunk winds up in your lungs.

SAY YES TO NO: NITRIC OXIDE IS
THE GAS THAT KEEPS GIVING

Inside your nose — in the paranasal sinuses, to be exact — you produce a gas called nitric oxide (NO). When you breathe through your nose, you draw NO into your body. When you breathe through your mouth, you do not. NO is pure magic for your health! For one thing, NO is a vasodilator, which means it widens blood vessels for easier flow and faster oxygen delivery. It's also a gasotransmitter, a gas that is an endocrine signaler, helping hormones like human growth hormone and insulin get their messages across.[21] Nitric oxide is an immunity sniper, picking off bacteria, viruses[22] (including coronaviruses[23]), fungi,[24] and free radicals.[25] When you breathe through the nose, air mingles with NO as it moves through your airways killing bugs, increasing oxygen uptake, and opening vessels for gangbuster pulmonary function.[26]

One way to increase natural production of NO is eating veggies that are high in nitrate. (FYI: Nitrate is not the same thing as sodium nitrate, a carcinogen found in highly processed foods.) It just so happens that nitrate-rich foods are also water rich (and hydrating) and full of antioxidants (reducing inflammation). These foods include celery, lettuce, spinach, beets, watercress, and arugula.[27] Antioxidant vitamins C and E and the supplement L-arginine, an essential amino acid, can also boost nitric oxide in the body.[28]

Since **low NO** can be a warning sign of heart problems and a cause of type 2 diabetes, it's a good idea to check your levels. You can get accurate readings with saliva test strips, which cost just pennies apiece and are available at pharmacies and online. I personally test my NO using Berkeley Life saliva test strips and can then use their supplement if my diet does not provide everything I need, usually when traveling. (Go to berkeleylife.com for more info.) **High NO** is a possible indication of asthma. A trip to a pulmonologist's office for a breath test, in which you exhale into a tube with a clip on your nose, can provide an accurate reading.

CONGESTION RX

Allergies, a cold or flu, and dry air can all cause clogged sinuses, aka congestion. If your nose is stuffed, what can you do but breathe through the mouth?

I have a friend who is slightly allergic to cats, but she loves her ragdoll Chonky too much to give her up. So congestion is just a part of her daily life. She mouth breathes whenever she's at home—especially at night when the cat is in the bed. Her partner came to me and begged for help. "I can't take the snoring," he said. "And her morning breath is so potent, it could kill our plants."

My advice was to keep the cat out of the bedroom, day and night (sorry, Chonky). Next, treat congestion with natural solutions that open airways and calm inflamed nasal tissues as a first step before seeing an allergist to talk about an OTC or prescription remedy.*

The same goes for anyone with a stuffy nose.

- **Nasal irrigation.** Use a neti pot (a small kettle-shaped vessel with a long spout) or a squeeze bottle to rinse your sinuses with a saline solution. The Federal Drug Administration approves this method[29] because it's safe and it works. First, clean the vessel. The last thing you want is to introduce bacteria or mold into your sinuses. Fill it with distilled or boiled (and cooled) water. Then follow the instructions on the packaging and add salt. Lean over the sink and tilt your head at a forty-five-degree angle. Place the end of the spout at the entrance of the upper nostril and pour in the saline solution. The solution will flush your sinus cavities, and then gush out of the bottom nostril, creating a weird sensation, to be sure. The salt does quick work to shrink inflamed tissues and clear airways for almost immediate relief.

- **Steam.** Inhaling steam reduces sinus pressure so mucus can drain. Take a shower, go into a steam room, or run hot water in the sink and lean over it with a towel over your head. My favorite method is boiling pasta. After I strain it, I

---

* If your congestion is chronic, it could be a sinus infection, nasal polyps, a deviated septum, or enlarged adenoids. It's worth a visit to an ENT doc to rule out such conditions.

put my face over the hot noodles. You get open airways and dinner at the same time.

- **Drink!** Hydration to the rescue again. Water intake won't instantly clear your nose, but well-hydrated mucus thins out and is easier to clear with other methods, such as using a neti pot or steam.
- **Ginger.** This root, in any form, is an anti-inflammatory powerhouse. Researchers put ginger extract up against an OTC antihistamine in a head-to-head competition to see which unclogged sinuses better. Five hundred ml of ginger extract was just as effective as the antihistamine, without the annoying side effects of drowsiness, fatigue, and constipation.[30] You can buy extract online or in health food stores. Just put a dropperful into water, and drink (follow the label for dosage instructions). Or you can cook with ginger, have ginger tea, or juice the root and do a shot.
- **Nasal dilators**. There are two types, external (think nasal strips) and internal, which are small things you put inside your nostril. I personally use internal ones (mutesnoring .com) for sleep and exercise, and they work great. Place nasal strips closer to the nostrils than to the bridge of the nose to get full advantage.

BREATHE CHANGE #2:
STRENGTHEN THE DIAPHRAGM

The diaphragm is a dome-shaped large muscle that sits below the lungs. It's the dividing line in the torso between the thoracic and abdominal regions. All day long, the diaphragm contracts (flattens) when you inhale to create suction that draws air into the lungs so they can fill up with O_2, and then relaxes (curves upward) when you exhale to create reverse pressure that empties the lungs of CO_2. The stronger your diaphragm, the more air you can take in and expel, for a robust, even heroic, gas exchange. The two layers of intercostal muscles of the rib cage are also engaged to allow the lungs to expand and contract.

Opera singers exercise their breathing muscles so they can hold notes longer and sound richer and fuller. My friend is a professional French horn player who has never exercised a day in his life. But when I gave him an at-home peak flow device—the one with the plastic balls in tubes that you blow into—he kept those balls aloft for five seconds on an inhale and six seconds on an exhale. It was truly humbling to see.

You don't need bulging biceps or quad muscles for super strong diaphragm and rib muscles. Nor do you need to break a sweat to exercise respiratory muscles.

Devices. Gizmos like the Airofit Pro, an **electronic mouthpiece** that measures peak airflow and lung capacity, train the lungs by using resistance, making it harder to inhale and exhale. It's like lifting weights, but for your respiratory muscles. It's effective, but expensive.

Endurance/elevation training masks fit over the nose and mouth. If used while exercising, these masks reduce airflow to lungs, so you have to work harder to breathe, increasing respiratory muscle strength. For around $30, you can buy an elevation training mask and fulfill your dream of looking like Bane in *The Dark Knight Rises*.

The inexpensive **low-tech options** are plastic tube-and-ball units. They do not use resistance to strengthen lung power. Improvement comes from repetition. I started with ten inhalations and ten exhalations per day on the device. At first, I could keep the balls up for two or three seconds. After two weeks of daily use, I was up to four seconds on each. It didn't take much time or effort to see significant improvement, just by blowing into a tube. My guess is that if I used a more technical device, I might progress a bit faster.

For intercostal flexibility and strength, try gate pose. You don't need expensive gadgets to improve your breathing strength. Start by kneeling with your knees hip-width apart, hands at your sides. Extend your left leg straight out to the side, keeping your pelvis squared. Lift your arms overhead, reaching for the sky. Then lean your upper body sideways over your left leg, facing forward. After a few seconds, straighten your torso and stretch both arms overhead. Return your left leg to kneeling, and switch sides.

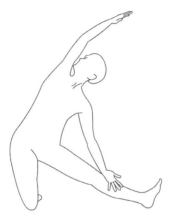

Side planks with torso twists (lift your free arm up into the air, then pivot to dip it under your body; return your arm to its original position and repeat) are also effective at working the intercostals.

To train the diaphragm, try belly breathing. Place your hand on your stomach, under the belly button, and breathe through the nose slowly, making your hand rise, and, without holding your breath, exhale slowly, engaging your core to draw your belly button toward the spine. (To make sure you aren't engaging the rib muscles, place the other hand over your heart. It should not move.) Do belly breathing for ten minutes, two or three times a day, and you'll notice a huge change in lung capacity very quickly. Side benefit: Toning the diaphragm tightens your abs.

BREATHE CHANGE #3:
STAND (AND SIT) TALL

Quick experiment:

- Sit in a chair and slouch forward, curving your spine. Place a hand on your stomach. Then inhale through the nose into the belly, making the hand rise.
- Sit up straight in the same chair with both feet planted on the floor. Hand on stomach, inhale through the nose into the belly, making the hand rise.

Which breath was deeper and easier? Which one lifted your hand more? Undoubtedly, you were able to inhale more deeply, for a longer count, when you sat up straight. It's simple mechanics. When you slouch, your lungs and other organs in your chest and abdomen are compressed. Your diaphragm is squished. There's just no room for much air. You're forced to take smaller breaths, with less oxygen, and short exhalations, expelling less cardon dioxide. The gas exchange process is stymied, and that triggers the stress response.

But when your back is straight and tall, your lungs can expand to capacity. Your diaphragm has the necessary space to flatten, creating the vacuum effect that draws in air. You inhale more O_2, and exhale more CO_2, super-charging the gas exchange to peak efficiency. When organs and tissues get the oxygen they need, you feel energized and calm.

Just like remembering to inhale and exhale through the nose, being mindful about your posture is one of the easiest ways to make a real impact on the quality of your breathing and, therefore, your state of body and mind.

If a gentle reminder to self to sit up straight isn't enough, try a posture corrector. They fall into two categories: (1) **strap-on braces or harnesses** that force the shoulders back and the chest out, and

(2) **electronic reminder devices** that you affix to your back between the shoulder blades that vibrate when you slouch. My daughter uses a posture reminder, and she loves it.

BREATHE CHANGE #4: CLEAR PHLEGM

It's completely normal to have phlegm (mucus). As you know, the slippery stuff is your best friend when it comes to trapping and killing bacteria that might otherwise cause an infection. However, excessive phlegm — due to smoking, a respiratory illness, being sedentary, aging — makes it difficult, even painful, to take deep, energizing, oxygenating breaths. Over time, uncleared phlegm can build up in your airways, limit lung capacity, and hinder gas exchange.

Better out than in. To help rid yourself of excess phlegm, cough. Coughing is the body's mechanism for moving phlegm and debris out of the lungs. It's not just for chest colds, though. You can use coughing techniques to dislodge mucus from the smaller bronchioles, and propel it through a bronchus, and finally up and out of the windpipe.

- **Controlled coughing**. Sit in a chair with your back straight and both feet planted on the floor. Inhale deeply through the nose into the belly. Hold the breath for two to four counts. Hinge forward slightly from the waist and cough sharply twice as you exhale. After breathing normally for a minute or two, repeat this process a few more times. You will know it's working if you feel something come up in the back of your throat.
- **Huff coughing**. Sit in a chair with the same straight back and planted feet. Inhale slowly into the abdomen

through the nose and hold for two or three seconds. When you exhale, make an O-shape with the lips and puff air quickly three times through the mouth while making a huff sound like you were trying to steam up a window.

Besides coughing, you can try supplementing. **Mullein**, a flowering plant, has been used as an herbal folk remedy for generations. The research shows that mullein is an effective anti-inflammatory[31] antibacterial powerhouse[32] and an expectorant (something that loosens phlegm, making it easier to cough up gunk). It's inexpensive and has no known side effects. When I tested liquid extract of mullein by putting an eyedropper's worth (1 ml) in my water bottle each day and engaged in controlled coughing, I moved a surprising amount of mucus from my airways. As always, follow the label for dosing instructions, and consult your doctor before taking any supplement, especially if you're pregnant or on prescription medication.

BREATHE CHANGE #5: MASTER THE TECHNIQUES

You've habituated nose breathing, gained respiratory muscle strength and flexibility, improved your posture, and cleared excess phlegm. Now you are ready to take breathing to the next level. For every situation in life, there is a breathing technique to learn and master. Starting with these:

Calming Breathing

Use calming techniques whenever you feel overwhelmed or anxious. Start with one minute of each method below and work your way up to ten minutes.

- **4-7-8.** Very simply, inhale into the belly for a count of four. Hold your breath gently for a count of seven. And then exhale slowly, drawing your belly in, for a count of eight. The entire cycle takes nineteen seconds, putting your respiratory rate at a very low and slow three cycles per minute. Your heart rate and blood pressure will decrease, and your stress response will switch off.
- **4-4-4-4, aka box breathing.** Inhale for a count of four, hold for four counts, exhale for four, hold for four. Each cycle lasts sixteen seconds, or a respiratory rate of around four cycles per minute. Guaranteed to calm you down quickly.
- **Alternate-nostril breathing, aka nadi shodhana pranayama.** This technique reduces stress and anxiety, lowers heart rate and blood pressure, and boosts memory and cognitive function.[33] A few variations to try: (1) Inhale through one nostril while holding the other closed, then exhale through the other. (2) Inhale and exhale through one nostril, then switch to the other side. (3) Inhale through one nostril, hold your breath, then exhale through the opposite or same nostril, then switch sides.
- **Cyclic or physiological sighing.** In 2023, researchers at Stanford School of Medicine published their research on cyclic sighing, a technique that boosts positive affect (feeling more joy), decreases heart rate, and switches on calm mode.[34] Given the emotional and physiological benefits, this method is surprisingly simple: Inhale through the nose deeply. On top of that, take another inhale until you can't take in any more air. Without holding your breath, slowly exhale through the mouth until all the air is out. Do it up to three times in a row when stressed for relief in under a minute. If you can build up

to a daily practice of five minutes per day, excellent! You'll enjoy better mood, sleep, focus, and emotional regulation. I have personally found this technique to be very effective.

Alertness Breathing

The following methods switch on the sympathetic nervous system to increase heart rate and send oxygen-rich blood to the brain to sharpen the mind and create a quick energy boost. It might seem counterintuitive to purposefully put yourself in fight-or-flight mode if the big picture goal is hormonal balance (meaning, less cortisol dominance). But by doing controlled hyperventilation, you can raise the bar for what switches on your stress response, so it won't happen on a hair trigger. Over time, these exercises will help you become a more relaxed, chill person who can handle difficult moments without stressing out.

- **Cyclic hyperventilation.** The Stanford team came up with this technique to speed up heart rate and trigger the release of adrenaline for insta-alertness and focus.[35] First, take a deep nasal inhale for a second or two, followed immediately by a fast mouth exhale. It's a one-two cycle, no holding, no counting. Repeat twenty-five times. Then, after the last inhale, exhale fully until you can't squeeze out any more air. Then hold your breath for fifteen to thirty seconds (use a stopwatch). Rapid breathing—hyperventilation—can be unsettling. You are purposefully triggering the stress response to get that quick hit of adrenal hormones that put you on high alert. You might get dizzy or feel tingling in the hands and feet (do not try this standing up). After a minute or two, the weirdness will stop, and you'll just feel sharper. Warning: This technique is not for people with an anxiety disorder. Only do it in a controlled, stable setting, never while driving or swimming.

- **Wim Hoff method**. Wim Hoff is a Dutch motivational speaker and extreme athlete, the man who brought ice bathing to the masses. His controlled hyperventilation method is very similar to the Stanford team's. Start by taking a deep belly breath through the nose or mouth, then passively exhale it. Repeat thirty times. On the final exhale, enter a "retention phase" of holding your breath for as long as you can, followed by a "recovery phase" of taking one more deep belly breath, holding it for fifteen seconds, and then letting it all go. Repeat three or four times. It's normal to feel lightheaded or tingly, and those symptoms will pass quickly.[36] If you combine Wim Hoff breathing with cold therapy (such as getting in an ice bath), it reduces one's perception of stress.[37] A few years ago, Wim Hoff trained my son and me in his breathing techniques prior to an ice bath.

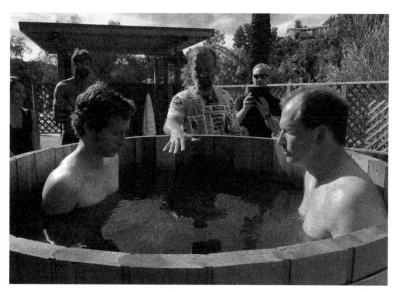

Cooper and me, sitting in ice water; Wim Hoff overseeing. I still remember the pain.

- **Laughter yoga.** Right now, smile big and go "ho-ho-ho, ha-ha-ha" as if you were really laughing at *Parks and Recreation*. Genuine amusement is not as important as making the sounds and breathing rapidly. The body doesn't care if laughter is fake. As long as you're laughing, oxygen intake goes up, and happy hormones like serotonin and dopamine are released, making you feel energized. A Turkish study of 101 nurses during the height of the pandemic found that laughter yoga helped this under-pressure group avoid burnout and feel greater life satisfaction.[38]

- **Skull-shining breath, aka kapalbhati.** Another controlled hyperventilation method, this yogic practice combines passive inhales with rapid, forceful exhales via snapping the belly inward. Start by sitting in a chair, hands on your thighs, back straight. Inhale through the nose and exhale sharply through the nose by contracting your abs. Inhaling will happen automatically if you keep snapping your belly inward to force the exhale, a fast pace of one belly snap per second. In yoga classes I've taken, instructors keep this up for two full minutes. Try it for thirty seconds at first and build as you get more comfortable.

- **Breath of fire, aka Agni Pran.** A Kundalini yoga method, breath of fire is another variation on rapid, rhythmic breathing. It's similar to skull-shining breath, but instead of inhaling and exhaling through the nose, breath of fire has you exhale through the mouth with a panting sound. Start by sitting with your back straight. Inhale into the nose until the belly rises, then snap your navel to force and exhale through the mouth, with a "heh" or panting sound. Repeat at a fast pace, one breath per second, for a minute. Work up to going longer as you feel more comfortable.

Appetite-Control Breathing

This method is not meant to reduce appetite to avoid meals. Deprivation diets do not work for weight loss, happiness, or anything else, except making yourself miserable when the diet inevitably proves unsuccessful. A plant-based, lean-protein diet, daily movement, good sleep, sufficient hydration, and mindful breathing are far safer and more effective strategies for weight loss. Use this breathing method to quiet hunger pangs between meals.

To take the edge off hunger:

- **Modified Qigong breathing**. Stand up with your feet shoulder-width apart. Place your hands right under your rib cage as a mental reminder to keep the air above that line. With squared shoulders, inhale into the chest with your belly pulled in. Hold the breath while keeping your abs tight. Then exhale, relaxing your upper body but keeping the abs engaged. Repeat ten times.

Sleep-Inducing Breathing

Deep rhythmic breathing is a relaxation technique that will calm your body and brain for sleep. But the breathe-sleep connection goes deeper than that. Diaphragmatic breathing is a treatment for sleep onset insomnia because:

It tones the vagus nerve and switches on rest-and-digest mode.

It promotes the production of melatonin, the sleepy hormone.[39]

It lowers heart rate and blood pressure to allow you to sleep.

When I'm working with Dolphin chronotypes, I recommend:

Resonant breathing. This is a variation on calming techniques with longer exhalations than inhalations. First of all, do this technique in bed when you're ready to sleep. Once you've lain down comfortably in bed, turn the lights out. Then, inhale for a count of four through the nose and exhale for a count of six. Repeat this cycle ten times. A British study found that ten minutes of daily resonant breathing sessions in this pattern helped long-COVID-19 patients reduce their symptoms, enjoy a higher quality of life, and get to sleep with greater ease.[40] If it works for them with their cluster of chronic conditions, it's worth a try for anyone.

OUR LIPS ARE SEALED . . . WITH TAPE

Per the American Academy of Sleep Medicine, your ability to breathe through the nose "plays an important role in the physiology of sleep." For anyone who sleeps with their mouth open, I recommend **mouth tape**, which is exactly what it sounds like. It's a strip of skin-friendly tape that fits over your lips, ensuring that your mouth stays closed overnight. A simple barrier can make a profound impact. You know all the benefits of nasal breathing already, nitric oxide magic, lowered stress, increased O_2 intake. Doing it overnight nets you more of that good stuff, along with preventing dental problems and bad breath. According to 2022 research, mouth tape is an effective alternative treatment for very mild OSA.[41] (If you are on a CPAP machine, consult your doctor before making any changes to your treatment.)

A middle-aged patient of mine, a man named Eric, struggled with anxiety-related insomnia. As soon as he got in bed, he would start to worry about not falling asleep, and that would spiral into a stress response as he lay in bed in the dark. His heart would start racing; his breathing became shallow and fast. In that physiological state, there was simply no way he could calm down enough to drift off.

I worked very closely with him on various treatments, like guided imagery and diaphragmatic breathing. Nothing worked. And then, almost as an aside, I suggested he try mouth tape.

I'll let Eric tell it: "It was uncomfortable at first to have tape on my mouth," he said. "I had to get used to that. But thinking about the tape was better than ruminating about everything that would go wrong if I didn't fall immediately asleep. When I did drift off, I was amazed to wake up seven hours later without having woken up once. I doubt I'd had three consecutive hours of sleep in years. I started using mouth tape every night, continue to be stunned months later."

Eric's anxiety panting in bed and his fitful, fragmented sleep triggered a stress response that aroused his body when he should have been simmering down. When he used mouth tape, the nasal breathing switched off stress mode, activated the parasympathetic nervous system, and allowed him, finally, to rest.

BREATHE CHANGE #6:
GET BLOOD MOVING

Oxygen and carbon dioxide are carried by hemoglobin, a protein in red blood cells. They deliver and remove those gasses via the bloodstream, aka your circulatory system. Without robust circulation, the entire point of respiration would be moot. Anything you do to benefit the circulatory system has a direct beneficial relationship with respiration. Here are examples:

Aerobic exercise. Cardio used to be more commonly called aerobic ("requiring oxygen") exercise because it forces you to draw in more oxygen at a faster pace than when you are resting or lightly exercising. When heart rate is increased but you can still hold a conversation, you're in the cardiorespiratory sweet spot.

Jump. When your watch tells you it's time to stand, actually do it. Every hour, get up and, for one minute, jump up and down. Bouncing movement gets your blood going because it speeds up the heart. It also energizes lymphatic fluid that relies on valves to keep moving.

Eat the good stuff. I don't have to tell you what that means. Fruits, veggies, whole grains, lean protein, healthy fats, whole foods. You know this by heart already. Fiber-rich, water-rich foods are great for hydration and circulation. Eat a plant or ten today.

Drink! Hydration = increased blood volume and circulation. Hit your hydration goals to keep your blood and the gas exchange cranking.

Quit or cut back on circulation blockers. Smoking causes respiratory havoc by introducing toxic tar and chemicals into your lungs, damaging airways, and clogging the system with sputum. Smoking is a wrecking ball for your circulatory system, too, damaging the heart and blood vessels. Alcohol isn't doing you any cardio-respiratory favors either. It depresses the central nervous system, affecting heart and lung function.

Breathing and Exercise FAQs

Should I breathe through the nose while exercising? It might feel more natural to breathe through the mouth when going hard on the track, field, or gym. The mouth is bigger, and you can take in more air volume that way. But volume isn't everything. Breathing effi-ciency—getting more oxygen in the system per breath—is just as or more important. And you do more with less if you breathe through the nose during moderate exercise. For long and steady exercise, like running a marathon, nasal breathing does a better job of sending oxygen where it needs to go for maximum benefit.[42] However, for short and intense exercise like sprinting, you need as much O_2 as possible. In that case, oral breathing might be the winner.

What is heart rate variability (HRV) and what does it have to do with breathing? HRV is the measure of time between heart-beats. The range of normal depends on age, sex, weight, and fitness

228

level. The normal range for adults is between 20 and 200 milliseconds. Having a high HRV—more time between beats—just means that your body is resilient and can adapt quickly to stress. A lower HRV, with relatively short time between beats, can mean that your autonomic nervous system is imbalanced, or that you're in chronic fight-or-flight stress mode. It can also be a sign of illness, dehydration, insufficient sleep, and being out of shape.

There are instances in life, however, when you intentionally want to activate the sympathetic nervous system. One of those times might be when you are playing sports. Get a competitive edge by "gaming" HRV with breathing techniques. Do so by choosing one of the Alertness Breathing techniques above to send blood to your muscles, get your heart going to give you a quick release of stress hormones, including vroom-vroom adrenaline.

HEART AND LUNG HELPERS

Anything that's good for the heart is also good for the lungs. So boost your breathing by consuming these heart-supporting foods and supplements (after consulting with your doctor):

- **Omega-3 fatty acids**. Eat a lot of SMASH fish (salmon, mackerel, anchovies, sardines, herring), or take omega-3s in capsules for anti-inflammatory and heart-healthy properties.
- **Coenzyme Q10 (CoQ10)**. An antioxidant, it boosts blood flow. Take it in pill form, or increase intake of fatty fish such as tuna and mackerel, organ meats such as liver, and whole grains.
- **L-Arginine**. Found in protein-rich foods. Inside the body, this amino acid turns into your BFF nitric oxide. (Not recommended for people who have recently had a heart attack, though.)
- **Garlic**. What's bad for vampires is great for the human heart. Garlic is anti-inflammatory and lowers blood pressure.

- **Cayenne pepper.** Found in spicy peppers, the "hot" compound capsaicin has anti-inflammatory qualities and can help lower blood pressure.
- **Ginkgo biloba** also helps widen blood vessels for healthy flow.
- **Turmeric.** An anti-inflammatory powerhouse. Any reduction in inflammation clears vessels and helps keep blood moving.
- **Antioxidants. Vitamins C and E** neutralize free radicals and keep oxidative stress and inflammation under control.
- **Magnesium.** It supports both the heart and the lungs and promotes sleep as well.
- **Vitamin D** boosts lung function.
- **N-Acetyl cysteine (NAC).** An amino acid derivative, it clears up excess phlegm.

Doing the Breathwork

Many people think breathwork and meditation are interchangeable. That's not true at all. During meditation, you might start by counting your normal breaths and concentrating on the rise and fall of your chest and belly. By focusing on one thing, you clear away extraneous thoughts and quiet the monkey mind to be present in the moment.

In breathwork, you focus on inhaling and exhaling, too, but the work is to intentionally alter your breathing patterns. By controlling the timing and duration of oxygen intake and carbon dioxide output, you can change your internal functioning. It's not primarily a mental exercise; it's physical.

Mindful breathing reduces stress as much as, if not more than, meditation, and in less time. Personally, I prefer to practice breathwork and follow it with meditation. The breathwork seems to bring me to a "present" state, and then I am open to the meditation.

Although lying on a yoga mat in a dimly lit room and breathing in time with loud, rhythmic music along with hundreds of other people seems like the wellness trend of the moment, the practice of breathwork—controlled breathing to evoke calm, emotional release, and spiritual insight—is not new. Yogis have been teaching pranayama breathing techniques to energize and mobilize the life force within since the practice developed in India thousands of years ago. You have done breathwork if you've ever taken a yoga class that included ujjayi (victorious breath, making a hissing or whispering sound in the back of the throat), simhasana (lion's breath, an invigorating practice in which you stick out your tongue while exhaling with a "haaa!" sound), or kapalbhati (breath of fire, snapping the abdomen for forced exhales and passive inhales).

There are popular workshops, often advertised on social media with clips of people weeping, shaking, and screaming, that can last two or three hours and claim to heal trauma through breathwork, promising that extended controlled breathing can clear the body of stored emotional trauma. Science does confirm breathwork's healing potential. For a 2023 Dutch study, participants did a forty-five-minute session of "connected breathwork," a guided intervention with fast diaphragmatic breathing. Researchers analyzed brain imaging before and after the workshop and found that cranial activity parameters shifted to "better mental condition." The researchers concluded that breathwork has "therapeutic benefits on a neuropsychological level."[43]

In a January 2024 *New York Times* article, the Czech-born American psychiatrist Stanislav Grof, who developed holotropic ("moving toward wholeness") breathing, was quoted claiming that doing breathwork could alter consciousness as much as psychedelic drugs do. The article paraphrases him, stating that altered states allow people to "unravel the root causes of their suffering quickly, making them more effective than conventional treatments like antidepressants."[44] The idea is that talk therapy is inherently limited because some hurts can't be expressed or resolved with words. But by breathing oneself into an altered state, it is possible to access buried trauma and purge yourself of it.

For people who have been doing an hour a week of talk therapy for years, the idea of doing a few hours of breathwork to change their minds for the better sounds fantastic. I'm not saying you should fire your shrink or flush your Zoloft, though. The science is still emerging, but breathwork looks to be another viable way to heal, gain insight, and find peace.*

> ***Air Awareness***: *In my men's group, we have daily breathwork and go on occasional retreats. On two of those trips, we did thirty minutes of guided hyperventilation work. I have to admit, I wish I had done it twenty years earlier. While it's very hard to describe, I can tell you that when it was over, I forgave some people in my life, who have also forgiven me. I know this sounds a little on the woo-woo side, but it's the truth. If I had known about breathwork like this early in my clinical career, I would have had everyone doing it.*

I've just given you a ton of information over the last twelve chapters. It's a lot. Don't worry about remembering everything or implementing all the advice on your own. The next section of the book is the **Sleep-Drink-Breathe Plan**, a three-week method for putting all the best practices for sleeping, drinking, and breathing

---

* Breathwork seminars or workshops are intense experiences and not appropriate or safe for anyone who has a respiratory illness, a heart condition, or seizures or is pregnant or underage.

together, with clear, easy-to-follow instructions. All you have to do is follow the daily recommendation three times a day to nudge the Dominos of Wellness. And then, once you get them down, all you have to do is sit back and watch your health goals fall into place.

But first, we'll take one last look at how the three Dominos of Wellness affect each other.

TAKEAWAYS

- Consciously improving breathing technique will earn you lower inflammation, more energy, and stronger immunity for a longer, healthier, and happier life.
- Plus, appetite control! Instant relaxation! Emotional regulation! Boosted circulation and detox! Better orgasms!
- Nose hairs and mucus aren't beloved by all. But they are the unsung heroes of infection prevention and healthy nasal breathing.
- By nose breathing (as opposed to mouth breathing), you take in more air, produce more nitric oxide, and enjoy a slew of other benefits.
- You can use specific breathing techniques for instant calm or instant energy, as needed. With practice, these methods will become second nature. You can use them whenever you need to either relax or become more alert.
- Forget leg day and arm day. Work a diaphragm day into your exercise routine. Strengthening the diaphragm leads to fuller and easier air intake. You can do it with deep belly breathing techniques or with air-resistance gizmos.
- Good posture is critical to good breathing. When sitting or standing, straighten up, with shoulders back and chest out for deeper inhalations and powerful exhalations.

- Breathwork can improve your lung capacity and perhaps help you resolve psychological trauma. Some experts believe it's better than talk therapy for emotional healing. It is certainly a useful technique for relaxation and enhanced physical and mental performance.

CHAPTER 13

The Sleep-Drink-Breathe Nexus

It's all connected.

Getting each of the big three Dominos of Wellness down improves your overall health in profound ways. I've shown you how getting better sleep, staying hydrated, and breathing properly helps you lose weight, reduce inflammation, and boost immunity and energy, among many other benefits. Wellness doesn't have to be elusive, or expensive, or complicated. It hinges on making simple changes that improve your most basic functions.

Pulling the lens back to see the bigger picture, I want to show you how knocking down one Domino of Wellness affects the other two, forward, backward, and sideways. Sleeping well leads to better hydration and breathing. Staying hydrated improves sleep and breathing. And breathing properly leads to better sleep and hydration.

The interconnectedness is so striking, it seems obvious our most elemental life-supporting systems evolved to work together to achieve the harmonious state of mind and body where everything is in homeostasis. The body wants to be well. When you improve one system, you improve the others, too. It works both ways, though. If one system isn't working, it causes glitches in the others, too.

I've been pointing out all along how sleeping, drinking, and breathing support each other. I'm going to lay it all out for you one more time, just to cement in your mind how real and impactful the domino theory of wellness is. If you already get it, then you can jump to page 241 to start the program!

THE SLEEP-DRINK NEXUS
How does sleep affect hydration?

- **Fluid loss**. Sleep incurs fluid loss via sweat and exhalation, and it's normal to wake up thirsty. If you follow the Sleep-Drink-Breathe Plan and drink 16 ounces of water after waking, you mitigate the water loss completely.
- **Hormonal balance**. Sleep and the kidney-regulating hormone work together to keep you from having to pee every few hours while asleep. But when sleep is disrupted or inadequate, the kidney rhythm can be thrown off, resulting in dehydration.
- **Loss of thirst**. A side effect of sleep deprivation is losing the sense of thirst. You don't know whether you need to drink, so you're less likely to do it.
- **Brain function**. During Stage 3 sleep and REM, the glymphatic system flushes out and detoxes the brain, including the area where your thirst and respiratory command centers and the master clock are located. So sleep reinforces thirst and respiratory drives, as well as chronorhythms that control every other system in the body.

THE DRINK-SLEEP NEXUS
How does hydration improve sleep?

- **Body temperature regulation**. When you sleep, body temperature goes down; it's a signal for melatonin release. When dehydrated, body temperature regulation goes haywire. Staying hydrated allows your body to cool down so that you can fall asleep.
- **Thinner mucus**. When you are well hydrated, the mucus in your airways thins, which helps clear sleep-disrupting nasal congestion. Thick mucus leads to snoring, which can disrupt sleep (and definitely makes you unpopular with a bed partner).
- **Fewer cramps**. Ever had a painful cramp in your calf or foot when you were trying to fall asleep, or woke up because of one? A chief cause of nighttime leg cramping is dehydration. Hitting your hydration goals can prevent cramps.
- **Hormonal balance**. A dehydrated body is under stress and therefore releases cortisol. Staying hydrated helps keep cortisol rhythm as it should be, lower at night and flowing at dawn to wake you up.
- **Less insomnia**. Although chronic insomnia may be due to your genetically determined chronotype (hello, Dolphins!), circumstantial acute insomnia is caused by stress. Stress can be mitigated by staying hydrated throughout the day.

THE SLEEP-BREATHE NEXUS
How does sleep affect breathing?

- **Respiratory rate**. During sleep, your respiratory rate changes. During non-REM sleep (Stages 1, 2, and 3), your rate is slower than during waking hours. A slow respiratory rate keeps you in calm mode, enabling rest. During dreamy REM sleep, your respiratory rate is almost the same as during wakefulness.

- **Sleep apnea.** Not a happy connection. This category of sleep disorders interrupts normal breathing overnight, which keeps you from getting adequate time in each sleep stage and leaves you sleep-deprived.

THE BREATHE-SLEEP NEXUS
How does breathing affect sleep?

- **Relaxation.** Deep belly breathing with longer exhalations than inhalations calms the body and mind so that you can drift off to sleep.
- **Cortisol shutoff.** For Dolphin chronotypes only: Your cortisol rhythm works in reverse, compared to Bears, Lions, and Wolves. When your stress hormone keeps flowing at night, you can game your system with deep diaphragm breathing techniques like 4-7-8 or box breathing to turn that cortisol trend around, allowing you to relax and quiet down physically and mentally for rest.

THE DRINK-BREATHE NEXUS
How does hydration affect breathing?

- **Slippery mucus.** Drink to keep your respiratory system's mucus layers viscous and slippery so air glides through while pathogens and pollutants get caught in the goo before they can become respiratory infections.
- **Airway flexibility.** Your trachea, bronchi, bronchioles, and alveoli are not made of wood. They are soft tissues. As you inhale and exhale, they need to expand and contract. Hydration keeps them supple.

- **Blood volume.** As you know, O_2 and CO_2 are toted around on red blood cells. You need a raging river of blood to move and exchange all that gas. To increase blood volume, drink!
- **Efficient O_2 uptake.** Your hungry cells need to be well hydrated to slurp up life-sustaining oxygen, use it to make energy, and then spit out the byproduct CO_2.

THE BREATHE-DRINK NEXUS
How does breathing affect hydration?

- **Moisture.** When you breathe through the nose of a well-hydrated body, the air is moist before it travels into the windpipe and lungs. That extra juiciness adds up to over 20,000 breaths in a day and prevents dehydration in the body as a whole. Mouth breathing has been found to incur 42 percent more water loss compared to nose breathing.[1]
- **Overall calm.** Deep belly breathing helps keep you calm and relaxed, which is beneficial for sleep, so that you are well rested enough to have a sensitive thirst drive.
- **Overall awareness.** Focusing on upright posture and deep breathing throughout the day makes you more aware of your body, which makes you more sensitive to your body's cues, like thirst.

Now that you've taken in twelve chapters of science, you have all you need to enact the Sleep-Drink-Breathe Plan. One last note — I know I've talked down expensive or high-pressure wellness routines and tools a bit in this book, but only to say that you don't *need* all the bells and whistles to create long-lasting healthy habits. I'm ultimately a big fan of green juices, I understand the motivation of a new gym outfit, and I've experienced transformations at expensive yoga and breathwork retreats. Once you have the basics down, there's no limit to how much you can supplement your wellness routine, with no judgment from me as to how you choose to motivate yourself to make smart choices! I hope this book has shown you that real wellness doesn't have a price tag and that it's accessible, actionable, and easy to start right now—where you go from here is up to you. So, on that note, the next pages will help you put all the information to good use and start knocking down those dominos. Let's go!

The Sleep-Drink-Breathe Plan

PREPARATIONS

WEEK 1

WEEK 2

WEEK 3

> *I've been promising you a simple plan to help you put all the foregoing information to use. If a plan is too complicated, no one will follow it or keep up with it for long. The Sleep-Drink-Breathe Plan is incredibly easy to follow and to incorporate into your life.*

You have probably noticed the dominos I've sprinkled throughout this book. They symbolize how optimizing the three Dominos of Wellness (the three dots on one side) can bring about whole-body balance (the one dot on the other side).

You may have noticed how much I love the number three.

The symbolism also applies to the Sleep-Drink-Breathe Plan. Over the next three weeks, for no more than one hour per day—with minimal effort and only optional expense—you will knock down the Dominos of Wellness and become a whole new person from the inside out. By doing so, you'll get the basics down and uncomplicate wellness—and it doesn't have to cost you a dime. As you improve the biobehaviors of sleep, hydration, and breathing, you'll soon notice that other healthy behaviors, and your wellness goals, will start falling into place on their own.

The Plan is organized weekly, so below, you'll find specific to-do's for Week 1, Week 2, and Week 3. Things start out slowly. At first, you'll incorporate only a few changes in your life at a time. And then you'll layer on a couple more, and so on. As you adapt to your new lifestyle, you'll notice improvement in energy and mood immediately, and that will keep you motivated to keep going. Not that any of the changes you make are hard or painful! They're all easy and pleasant, as you'll see. In fact, you will come to look forward to every action item in this plan and maybe even feel weird if you don't do it.

TIMING IS EVERYTHING

There's another important number in this plan: five. Five times per day, you will tend to your Dominos. Those five times are:

- **Upon waking**. The start of your day, and the first opportunity to knock down some dominos for Big D(ay) Energy.
- **Mid-morning**. Sleep inertia has faded, and the day is underway. Tending to your Dominos now will keep your energy, mood, and concentration up.
- **Post-Lunch**. Typically, people feel an afternoon energy lag one or two hours after the midday meal, called the postprandial dip. Domino tasks can revive you.

- **Pre-Dinner.** Domino tasks at this time can give you a second wind if you're going out or help you unwind after a long day.
- **Pre-Bedtime.** Set yourself up for a great night ahead. Three hours before bed: last call for alcohol, caffeine, nicotine, food, and exercise (unless you're a Wolf). Two hours before bedtime: last call for water. One hour before bed: Begin the Power-Down Hour, offscreen deceleration, and relaxation before sleep.

These five daily Domino times are important because they correspond with the ebbs and flows of your circadian rhythms. Each chronotype has its own chronorhythm. I will tell you exactly what to do during each of these times in just a bit. For now, confirm your chronotype at chronoquiz.com if you haven't already done so.

	Bear	Lion	Wolf	Dolphin
Upon Waking	7:00 a.m.	6:00 a.m.	8:00 a.m.	6:30 a.m.
Mid-Morning	10:00 a.m.	9:00 a.m.	11:00 a.m.	9:30 a.m.
Post-Lunch	2:00 p.m.	1:00 p.m.	3:00 p.m.	3:00 p.m.
Pre-Dinner	6:00 p.m.	5:00 p.m.	7:00 p.m.	6:30 p.m.
Pre-Bedtime Countdown Begins at...	8:00 p.m.	7:00 p.m.	9:00 p.m.	9:00 p.m.

To Do Right Now: Set five alarms on your phone or watch at the corresponding times for your chronotype. To set alarms on Apple and Android devices, go to the clock app, and then go to alarms. Input the time, and you will be prompted to repeat. Choose to repeat every day.

PREPARATION IS EVERYTHING, TOO

Before you start the plan, there are just two prep tasks to take care of first.

Rehab Your Bedroom

Make it clean and cozy. If your sheets are ancient, it's time for an upgrade. If your pillows and mattress are old and saggy, invest in your sleep and health by getting new ones. I've made this a bit easier with over 150 reviews on my website (sleepdoctor.com).

Your bedroom is for sleep (and sex) only. It shouldn't be a dining room, living room, or playroom. So take an hour or two to rearrange things (you may need to move a desk, work materials, kids' toys, dirty dishes, etc., out of there). While you're at it, unclutter the space and neaten it up. The fewer distractions, like piles of laundry, your laptop, a stack of bills, the better it will be for sleep.

Dark, cool, quiet, and humid. Once your bedroom has been stripped of distractions and things that remind you of your waking life, make it even more slumber friendly. Do you have blinds or curtains on the windows? If not, order a good eye mask to block light. Same goes for an air conditioner if you live in a warm climate. The room should be kept at 65 to 70 degrees at night. If noise is an issue, order earplugs or a white noise machine. If you live in a dry climate, use a humidifier to reach the desired 30 to 50 percent humidity for sleep.

Other SDB Plan Supplies

The beauty of the Sleep-Drink-Breathe Plan is that you don't need to buy anything to do it. But some items can help and are worthwhile investments in your health.

For sleep. In the previous section, I recommended some sleep enhancers, such as an eye mask and earplugs, both very affordable.

If snoring (your own or your partner's) is an issue, you can buy mouth tape and see how that goes for you (as long as you have been tested for apnea). Sleep-supporting melatonin and magnesium supplements have no side effects if used correctly and can help people with sleep-onset and sleep-maintenance insomnia. (We sell excellent capsules and gummies at shop.sleepdoctor.com.) The big-ticket item in this category is an electronic sleep tracker that you wear on your wrist, finger, or forehead. My personal choice is an Oura ring. I like the form factor of a ring and you can get better data that way. Do your research, and if you decide not to buy an electronic sleep tracker, no problem! You will keep a low-tech sleep diary in any case for data collection.

For hydration. Only two items you might need to purchase in this category: a stainless steel or glass water bottle and a tap water filter.

For breathing. You absolutely do not need to buy such breath training equipment as a peak flow device, an endurance mask, or an oral gizmo like an Airofit trainer—but it's worth exploring what's out there if your lung capacity is limited or your diaphragm muscle is weak. Posture correctors such as harnesses or electronic signaling devices can help condition you to sit and stand up straight. Mouth tape will keep you breathing through the nose overnight. And mullein supplements (tincture or capsules) can help clear excess mucus from airways.

> **If you buy just one thing**: Get a decent tap water filter. You will love the change in taste, and that alone will inspire you to drink more. Just knowing that my water is clean motivates me to keep sipping.

Pre-Plan Self-Testing

You need to know where you started to see how far you've come. So I'm recommending that you do some of the at-home assessments to get baseline data before you begin the plan.

For sleep. If you wear a tracker, you are already collecting data about your sleep habits. You will notice improvement as you

SLEEP DIARY							
	M	T	W	Th	F	S	Su
I went to bed at...							
I fell asleep at...							
I woke up ___ times in the night...							
I woke up at...							
I snoozed the alarm ___ times...							
I got out of bed at...							
I had ___ caffeinated drinks...							
I had ___ alcoholic drinks...							
I napped for...							
I exercised for...							

progress through the plan. I recommend that everyone start keeping a pen-and-paper sleep diary to collect data about sleep quality and quantity and to track how alcohol, exercise, and medications affect sleep. You will make daily updates in your sleep diary throughout the three weeks of the plan.

For hydration. You don't have to count ounces of water intake because the plan takes care of that for you. It gets you to 64 ounces per day. And if you drink at least one 8-ounce serving of water at mealtimes as well, you will effortlessly hit a minimum of 88 ounces every day. For the three weeks of the plan, update a hydration diary at each of the five key times per day. You will assess two metrics: urine color and skin turgor (via the pinch test on page 113). The purpose is to make sure you are meeting hydration goals as you go through the day. If nothing more, it will remind you to drink. Here's a template you can use:

	Upon Waking	Mid-Morning	Post-Lunch	Pre-Dinner	Pre-Bedtime
Urine Color	clear				
Skin Turgor Test	Snapped back < 1 second				

And one last hydration baseline measure: I'd like you to take a "before" photo of your face first thing in the morning, no makeup or moisturizer. After three weeks, you'll take another photo and compare the two.

For breathing. The day before you start the Sleep-Drink-Breathe Plan, do the following tests (full descriptions start on page 178), and write down your results. You will retest all these metrics after three weeks.

My pre-SDB Plan respiratory rate: _____

My pre-SDB Plan shortness of breath rating: _____

Pre-SDB Plan, I can hold my breath for: _____

Once you have turned your bedroom into a sleep sanctuary and purchased whichever items you want to support your domino work, you are ready to begin knocking them down.

So let's get started.

WEEK 1

*Start Knocking Down Dominos with
Simple Tasks Five Times per Day*

During the first week, get used to the new routine.

UPON WAKING

Start the day well.

> Bear: 7:00 a.m.
> Lion: 6:00 a.m.
> Wolf: 8:00 a.m.
> Dolphin: 6:30 a.m.

Sleep To-Do's

- Get up when the alarm goes off. Do not snooze. You are going for consistency with your wake time! Very important.
- If the sun is up, go outside and get fifteen minutes of sunlight. This will signal to your master clock that the day has begun and that it's time to be fully awake. During winter, if the sun isn't out yet, grab time in the sun as soon as you can. If you live in a cloudy environment, consider buying full-spectrum light bulbs or a light box to get that morning boost.
- Input morning data into your sleep diary.

Drink To-Do's

- Sip 16 ounces of water, about an ounce per swallow.
- Check morning urine color and skin turgor and input the data in your hydration diary.

Breathe To-Do

Take fifteen deep breaths. The simplest technique: Inhale for four counts, extending the belly, and then exhale for four counts, drawing the belly button toward the spine. Imagine your inhalation sends air to every nook and cranny of your lungs. Every exhalation fully empties them.

MID-MORNING

Keep the wellness going.

Bear: 10:00 a.m.

Lion: 9:00 a.m.

Wolf: 11:00 a.m.

Dolphin: 9:30 a.m.

Sleep To-Do

Have one or two 8-ounce servings of caffeinated coffee or tea to slow down your sleep drive. Now that morning cortisol and adrenaline have faded, you can use the adenosine blocker in caffeine to keep up energy and concentration for the rest of the morning.

Drink To-Do's

- Coffee and tea count toward hydration. If you have only one cup, have another 8 ounces of plain water or unflavored seltzer for a total fluid intake of 16 ounces.
- Input mid-morning urine color and skin turgor data into your hydration diary.

Breathe To-Do

Take fifteen deep breaths. This week, stick to the most basic techniques. While seated, practice **4-4-4-4 box breathing**. Inhale for a count of four; hold for four; exhale for four; hold for four. Repeat another fourteen times.

POST-LUNCH

Ward off the postprandial dip.

Bear: 2:00 p.m.
Lion: 1:00 p.m.
Wolf: 3:00 p.m.
Dolphin: 3:00 p.m.

Sleep To-Do's

- Go outside for another fifteen minutes of sun to remind the master clock it's still daytime.
- Move a little. Boost your circulation (which is also great for hydration and breathing) by taking a walk around the block. Daytime movement enhances sleep later. Even five or ten minutes makes an impact.

Drink To-Do's

- Sip 16 ounces of plain water, herbal tea, or unflavored seltzer.
- Input urine color and skin turgor data into your hydration diary.

Breathe To-Do's

- If you are flagging, practice **cyclic hyperventilation**, an alertness breath technique: First, take a deep nasal inhalation for a second or two, followed immediately by a fast mouth exhalation. It's a quick one-two cycle, no holding, no counting. Repeat twenty-five times and then, after the last inhalation, exhale fully until you can't squeeze out any more air. Then hold your breath for fifteen to thirty seconds (use a stopwatch).
- If you are inappropriately hungry (you have a healthy lunch, but are craving quick-energy food anyway), try a

modified Qigong appetite-control breathing technique: With squared shoulders, inhale into the chest with your belly pulled in. Hold the breath while keeping your abs tight. Then exhale, relaxing your upper body but keeping the abs engaged. Repeat ten times.

PRE-DINNER

The night is young and you are well.

Bear: 6:00 p.m.
Lion: 5:00 p.m.
Wolf: 7:00 p.m.
Dolphin: 6:30 p.m.

Sleep To-Do's
- Prepare a meal with at least two servings of water-rich vegetables and fruit.
- Reinforce your master clock by finishing your dinner within four hours of bedtime.

Drink To-Do's
- Sip 16 ounces of room-temperature water a half-hour before eating. This will get your thermogenesis fires stoked, so you'll consume less at dinner and burn additional fat.
- Input urine color and skin turgor info into your hydration diary.

Breathe To-Do's
- Are you staying home tonight with minimal focus and concentration needs as you wind down? If so, take fifteen calming breaths. To keep it simple, stick with **box breathing**.

- Or do you intend to spend the next few hours finishing up some work or going out to socialize with friends? In that case, do a round of **cyclic hyperventilation** for an alertness boost.

PRE-BEDTIME

Set yourself up for a great night.

Count backward from...
Bear: 11:00 p.m.
Lion: 10:00 p.m.
Wolf: midnight
Dolphin: midnight

Three Hours Before Bed

For all chronotypes: Last call for alcohol, caffeine, nicotine, and food. Wolves can exercise, but no intense movement for anyone else.

Two Hours Before Bed

Last call for water. Sip 16 ounces of plain water or herbal tea.

One Hour Before Bed: Power-Down Hour

Sleep To-Do's

- Turn off electronics. That means no screens. Dim the lights. Darkness reinforces your circadian rhythm and tells your master clock that it's time for sleep.
- Don't engage in anything mentally stimulating. So don't read an addicting book. Bedtime reading should be a bit dry and dull. I'm a big fan of journaling before bed, as long as it's not going to wind you up.

- Quiet the body by taking a hot bath or shower or doing light stretching.
- Fill out the nighttime info in your sleep diary.

Drink To-Do's

- Refill your bedside water bottle so it's ready to go for your upon-waking intake.
- Do your final hydration diary entry of the day.

Breathe To-Do

Take fifteen deep, calming, sleepiness-inducing breaths. This week, practice **4-7-8 breathing** to quiet the nervous system so you can ease into sleep: Inhale into the belly for a count of four. Hold your breath gently for a count of seven. And then exhale slowly, drawing the belly in, for eight counts.

WEEK 2

*Continue Knocking Down Dominos with
Simple Tasks Five Times per Day*

During the second week, try some new strategies.

UPON WAKING

Start the day well.

Bear: 7:00 a.m.
Lion: 6:00 a.m.
Wolf: 8:00 a.m.
Dolphin: 6:30 a.m.

Sleep To-Do's

- Get up when the alarm goes off. Do not snooze. Pop out of bed, even if you are still tired.
- Get fifteen minutes of sunlight to signal to the master clock, "It's daytime now."
- Input morning data into your sleep diary.
- *NEW this week: Morning exercise people, if possible, do your workout outside for more of that circadian-reinforcing sunshine. Movement boosts circulation and helps with sleep later.*

Drink To-Do's

- Sip 16 ounces of water.
- Input urine color and skin turgor into your hydration diary.
- *NEW this week: If you work out in the morning, remember to drink an additional 12 ounces per thirty minutes of exercise.*

Breathe To-Do's

- Take fifteen deep breaths with a four-count inhalation into the belly, no hold, and a four-count exhalation.
- *NEW this week: Do a round of controlled coughing to wake up your lungs and clear away any excess mucus. Sit in a chair with your back straight and both feet planted on the floor. Inhale deeply through the nose into the belly. Hold the breath for two to four counts. Hinge forward slightly from the waist and cough sharply twice as you exhale.*

MID-MORNING

Keep the wellness going.

Bear: 10:00 a.m.

Lion: 9:00 a.m.

Wolf: 11:00 a.m.

Dolphin: 9:30 a.m.

Sleep To-Do

Have one or two 8-ounce servings of caffeinated coffee or tea to slow down your sleep drive.

Drink To-Do's

- If you have only one cup of coffee or tea, have another 8-ounce serving of plain water or unflavored seltzer now for a total fluid intake of 16 ounces.
- Input mid-morning urine color and skin turgor data into your hydration diary.

Breathe To-Do

Since you perfected box breathing last week, try a new technique, **cyclic sighing**, this week for a mid-morning boost of joy, clarity, and calm. Inhale through the nose deeply. On top of that, take another inhalation until you can't take in any more air. Without holding your breath, slowing exhale through the mouth until all the air is out. Repeat several times.

POST-LUNCH

Ward off the postprandial dip.

Bear: 2:00 p.m.
Lion: 1:00 p.m.
Wolf: 3:00 p.m.
Dolphin: 3:00 p.m.

Sleep To-Do's

- Grab ten to fifteen minutes of sunlight.
- Move a little to boost circulation. Again, don't go crazy. A short walk. A little dance. A few sun salutations.

Drink To-Do's

- Sip 16 ounces of plain water, herbal tea, or unflavored seltzer.
- Input data into your hydration diary.
- *NEW this week: Habits are formed if you enjoy doing them. Come up with two pleasurable activities you can link with your afternoon hydration practice. Perhaps chatting with a friend or doing a crossword puzzle.*

Breathe To-Do's

- If you are flagging, practice an alertness breathing technique like **cyclic hyperventilation** or **skull-shining breath**. Sit in a chair, hands on your thighs, back straight. Inhale through the nose, and exhale sharply through the nose by quickly contracting your abs. One breath per second. Try to keep going for a full minute.

- Or, if you are inappropriately hungry, try **modified Qigong** appetite-control breathing.
- *NEW this week: Practice posture awareness. Are you slouching? Mindfully straighten your back. Imagine a string is pulling your head up toward the ceiling.*

PRE-DINNER

The night is young and you are well.

Bear: 6:00 p.m.
Lion: 5:00 p.m.
Wolf: 7:00 p.m.
Dolphin: 6:30 p.m.

Sleep To-Do's

- Prepare a meal with at least two servings of water-rich veggies and fruit.
- Reinforce your master clock by finishing dinner within four hours of bedtime.
- *NEW this week: For some, morning movement isn't possible. So, for evening exercisers, make sure you complete your workout within three or, better, four hours before bedtime. Ideally, exercise before your final meal. Working out on a full stomach can cause digestive issues that may affect sleep later.*

Drink To-Do's

- To get your thermogenesis fires stoked, sip 16 ounces of room-temperature water a half-hour before eating.
- Input urine color and skin turgor info into your hydration diary.

- *NEW this week: If you exercised before dinner, remember to drink an additional 12 ounces for every thirty minutes of working out.*

Breathe To-Do's

- For a chill night, try a new calming technique, **alternate-nostril breathing**. Inhale through one nostril while holding the other closed, then exhale through the other. OR inhale and exhale through one nostril, then switch sides. OR inhale through one nostril, hold your breath, then exhale through the opposite or same nostril before switching sides.
- Or if you need your brain for work or to recharge your social battery for a night out, practice **cyclic hyperventilation** or **skull-shining breath**.
- *NEW this week: Evening posture check! How's your back doing? Even on the couch while watching TV, try to keep your shoulders back to create space for your lungs.*

PRE-BEDTIME

Set yourself up for a great night.

Count backward from ...
Bear: 11:00 p.m.
Lion: 10:00 p.m.
Wolf: midnight
Dolphin: midnight

Three Hours Before Bed

For all chronotypes: Last call for alcohol, caffeine, nicotine, and food. Wolves can exercise, but no intense exercise for anyone else.

Two Hours Before Bed

- Last call for water. Sip 16 ounces of plain water or herbal tea.
- *NEW this week: Come up with two good ideas of pleasant behaviors you can link with your final hydration of the night. Perhaps "tea and TV" or "sip and stretch."*

One Hour Before Bed: Power-Down Hour

Sleep To-Do's

- Turn off the TV, phones, laptops, and tablets. Even if you turn the brightness all the way down, the light can still confuse your master clock.
- Fill out the nighttime info in your sleep diary.
- Hot bath or shower, check. Light stretching, check.
- Don't set your brain on spinout. Avoid intense conversations. Don't sit down right before bed and examine your finances. This is not the right moment to tell your partner or child, "We need to talk." No movies with explosions or books about dragons. Listen to a meditation app or a pleasant, maybe slightly boring audiobook.
- *NEW this week: Practice acceptance if sleep doesn't come immediately. You are learning how to sleep well—and how to tolerate not sleeping well.*

Drink To-Do's

- Refill your bedside water bottle so it's ready to go for your upon-waking intake.
- Do your final hydration diary entry of the day.

Breathe To-Do's

- Try a new sleep breathing technique, **resonant breathing**. Start this technique at the end of Power-Down Hour, when you are ready to get in bed. Inhale for a count of four through the nose and exhale for a count of six through the nose. Repeat this cycle ten times.

- *NEW this week: Try mouth tape to prevent overnight mouth breathing.*

WEEK 3

*Benefit from Knocking Down Dominos with
Simple Tasks Five Times per Day.*

During the third week, try some advanced techniques.

UPON WAKING

Start the day well.

Bear: 7:00 a.m.
Lion: 6:00 a.m.
Wolf: 8:00 a.m.
Dolphin: 6:30 a.m.

Sleep To-Do's

- Get up when the alarm goes off. By now, you might not need that alarm.
- Get fifteen minutes of sunlight.
- Input morning data into your sleep diary.
- Morning exercise people, work out outside if possible.
- *NEW this week: At the end of your shower, blast cold water and stand under it for as long as you can. This will clear any sleep inertia and boost circulation.*

Drink To-Do's

- Sip 16 ounces of water.
- Input urine color and skin turgor into your hydration diary.
- If you worked out, remember to drink 12 ounces per thirty minutes of exercise.

- *NEW this week: On the last day of the last week of the plan, take a morning selfie, no makeup, no moisturizer. This is your "after" photo.*

Breathe To-Do's

- Take fifteen deep breaths. Inhale for four counts into the belly; no hold; exhale for four counts.
- Do a round of controlled coughing.
- *NEW this week: Strengthen your intercostal muscles by doing three rounds of side planks or gate pose. For gate pose, kneel with knees hip-width apart, hands at your sides. Extend your right leg straight out to the side, keeping your pelvis squared. Lift your arms overhead, reaching for the sky. Then lean your upper body over your right leg, facing forward. After a few seconds, straighten your torso and stretch both arms overhead. Return your right leg to kneeling, and switch sides.*

MID-MORNING

Keep the wellness going.

Bear: 10:00 a.m.
Lion: 9:00 a.m.
Wolf: 11:00 a.m.
Dolphin: 9:30 a.m.

Sleep To-Do's

- Have one or two 8-ounce servings of caffeinated coffee or tea to slow down your sleep drive.
- *NEW this week: Grab another blast of sun, even if you just stick your head out of the window. Move a bit. Any additional steps you take now will help you sleep later.*

Drink To-Do's

- If you have only one cup of coffee or tea, have another 8-ounce serving of plain water or unflavored seltzer.
- Input urine color and skin turgor data into your hydration diary.

Breathe To-Do's

- By now, you are a pro at **box breathing, cyclic hyperventilation, cyclic sighing,** and **skull-shining breath**. Choose your favorite technique or try **laughter yoga**. Smile big and go "ho-ho-ho, ha-ha-ha" as if you are really laughing. You might feel ridiculous, but your body doesn't know you're faking. You'll increase oxygen intake and get a hit of serotonin.
- *NEW this week: screen apnea check. While working at the computer, pause occasionally to check if you are holding your breath. If so, get up and move a bit to replenish lost oxygen intake.*
- *NEW this week: nose breathing check. As the alarm goes off to remind you to drink and breathe, check if your mouth is open.*

POST-LUNCH

Ward off the postprandial dip.

Bear: 2:00 p.m.
Lion: 1:00 p.m.
Wolf: 3:00 p.m.
Dolphin 3:00 p.m.

Sleep To-Do's

- Grab ten to fifteen minutes of sunlight.

- Move a little to boost circulation. Again, don't go crazy. A short walk. A little dance. A few sun salutations.
- *NEW this week: Bears and Lions, experiment with napping. Find a safe, quiet place to put your head down for up to thirty minutes. To avoid sleep inertia upon waking, Nap-a-Latte. Right before your nap, drink a cup of coffee. The caffeine will kick in twenty or thirty minutes later, right when you've planned to wake up, and erase any trace of grogginess. You'll be restored, clear-headed, and ready to go.*

Drink To-Do's

- Sip 16 ounces of water *while doing a pleasurable activity.*
- Input data into your hydration diary.
- *NEW this week: Taste test mineral water brands. Thus far, you've been drinking plain water, herbal tea, and seltzer. Drinking mineral water once or twice a day improves digestion and increases electrolytes. Try three brands and choose your favorite. Or make your own (recipe on page 156).*

Breathe To-Do's

- If you are flagging, practice an alertness breathing technique like **cyclic hyperventilation** or **skull-shining breath**.
- Or, if you are inappropriately hungry, try **modified Qigong** appetite-control breathing.
- Posture check.
- Screen apnea check.
- Nose breathing check.

PRE-DINNER

The night is young and you are well.

Bear: 6:00 p.m.
Lion: 5:00 p.m.
Wolf: 7:00 p.m.
Dolphin: 6:30 p.m.

Sleep To-Do's

- Prepare a meal with at least two servings of water-rich veggies and fruit.
- Reinforce your master clock by finishing dinner within four hours of bedtime.
- Evening workout. Shoot for completing it within four hours of bedtime. And, as always, do it before you eat so you don't have issues later.

Drink To-Do's

- Sip 16 ounces of room-temperature water a half-hour before eating.
- Input urine color and skin turgor info into your hydration diary.
- If you exercised before dinner, drink 12 ounces for every thirty minutes of working out.

Breathe To-Do's

- For a chill night, do a round of **alternate-nostril breathing**.
- Or if you need your brain for work or to recharge your social battery for a night out, practice **cyclic hyperventilation** or **skull-shining breath**.
- Evening posture check!

- *NEW this week: Heat. If you have access to a sauna, steam room, or infrared sauna blanket, use it for up to ten minutes to speed up circulation and gas exchange and boost detox. Not a daily activity, though. Do it two or three times per week, and hydrate afterward.*

PRE-BEDTIME

Set yourself up for a great night.

Count backward from . . .
Bear: 11:00 p.m.
Lion: 10:00 p.m.
Wolf: midnight
Dolphin: midnight

Three Hours Before Bed

For all chronotypes: Last call for alcohol, caffeine, nicotine, and food. Wolves can exercise, but no intense exercise for anyone else.

Two Hours Before Bed

Last call for water. Sip 16 ounces of plain water or herbal tea *while doing a pleasurable activity.*

One Hour Before Bed: Power-Down Hour

Sleep To-Do's

- Turn off electronics.
- Fill out the nighttime info in your sleep diary.
- Hot bath or shower, check. Light stretching, check.
- Avoid conflict and tension.
- Practice sleep acceptance. Whatever happens, happens. It's okay.

Drink To-Do's

- Refill your bedside water bottle so it's ready to go for your upon-waking intake.
- Do your final hydration diary entry of the day.

Breathe To-Do's

- Practice the calming breath method of your choice, **4-7-8 breathing, resonant breathing,** or **box breathing.**
- Have your mouth tape ready to go.

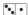

At the end of three weeks...

Your pants will feel looser.

Your poops will be magnificent.

You will feel more in control of your emotions, even during stressful times.

Inflammation-related aches and pains, such as headaches and joint pain, will be reduced.

Your moods will be more stable, and you'll feel more positive affect (a joyful outlook) about your life in general.

It feels like magic, but the results of doing the plan are due to pure science. Simply by prioritizing—and optimizing—sleep, hydration, and breathing, you can transform your health from the inside out.

HOW FAR YOU'VE COME

Compare your sleep data pre- and post-plan. Along with proof that you are sleeping solidly with fewer wake-ups, I want to draw your attention to any changes in alcohol intake and exercise. Because of the plan's last call for alcohol and recommendations for exercise, you have been drinking less and moving more.

Check changes in your daily number of steps. Since you have been taking two or three outdoor movement breaks throughout the day, your step counts have probably increased significantly.

Check your skin. Compare your no-makeup selfies at the beginning and end of the plan. With all that exercise, fresh air, and hydration, you will look fresher and more glowy than when you started. How's your expression? Perkier? Happier? Does your face look slimmer? I bet it does.

Check your breathing. Besides the measurable stats below, there are other indications that breathing techniques are working for you. Do you have less back, neck, and shoulder pain, due to posture awareness? Is your throat less dry and sore when you wake, due to mouth taping? Your morning breath will be better.

My post-SDB Plan respiratory rate: _____

My post-SDB Plan shortness of breath rating: _____

Post-SDB Plan, I can hold my breath for: _____

Perhaps the best change of all is that you just feel better. You are being proactive about your wellness by knocking down dominos, setting off a chain reaction that leads to improved health.

acknowledgments

Valerie Frankel: What a great experience this one has been. Thank you for reaching into my head and helping to pull out the simplicity of wellness. I value you and having you in my life. Thank you.

Tracy Behar: I can't thank you enough for having faith in our third project together. While I know you are now in a new world, I still value you and how you have always made me "want to write a better book." Thank you, T!

PR Team at Spark: Jess and Jules—what can I say—this time will be a bit more fun for sure!!!

Alex Glass: Dude, you are literally the best one out there. I talk to people all the time about their agents, I hear the horror stories—it's bad. Never with you. Your integrity, intelligence, and persistence are much appreciated. Also talking me off the ledge on occasion is certainly helpful!

Maggie Rosenberg: Thank you so much for your awesome illustrations.

Everyone at Little, Brown: Thank you for honoring me with faith in my work. I do not take that commitment lightly. I will show my gratitude by helping get this book into the hands of as many people as I possibly can.

Becky Johnston: Another one down: What can I say? It's still true: Everyone who meets you sings your praises, and let me tell you, they are correct. I could never help as many people as we do without your help. Thanks for being there.

Graham Purdy, JD Esq. at Hertz, Lichtenstein, Young, and Polk: Graham, YOU ROCK. I honestly think of you as my legal friend, more than as my lawyer. Your humor, kindness, integrity, and attention to detail are fantastic. I can't thank you enough for helping during the hard times.

Mickey Beyer Clausen: I still swear we are brothers. Someone told me that I am the average of my five closest friends; you are in the top five, for sure. Thank you for everything.

Joe Polish: You inspired a big part of this book (actually most of it). Thank you for teaching me the theory of Dominos, and thank you for continuing to be a part of my life.

All the amazing scientists who have contributed to the science of sleep, hydration, and breathwork. Without you, this book would never have been written. I am excited to get it to the masses and help them. Your work is cited in the Notes, and we want to thank every one of you for your contribution and acknowledge all your efforts to help make this book possible.

To my business partners who have helped in so many ways:

OneCare: Patrick, Bill, Keith, Raf, Jeff, Jeff, Holland, David, Colin, and Shan. While at times it certainly feels like Mr. Toad's Wild Ride, I want to thank each of you for making my dream come true.

Humanaut: To Paul and the team, I'm very excited for the future!

Steve Aoki: Bro, Pokémon, Thanksgiving, and your Mom's cookin'. This year Carson wants to jump off the roof!

notes

Introduction

1. National Sleep Foundation. *National Sleep Foundation's 2023 Sleep in America Poll*. 2023 March 9. https://www.thensf.org/wp-content/uploads/2023/03/NSF-2023-Sleep-in-America-Poll-Report.pdf.
2. Taylor K, Jones EB. Adult Dehydration. Treasure Island (FL): *StatPearls* Publishing; 2022 Oct. https://www.ncbi.nlm.nih.gov/books/NBK555956.
3. Thomas ET, Guppy M, Straus SE, et al. Rate of normal lung function decline in ageing adults: a systematic review of prospective cohort studies. *BMJ Open* 2019;9:e028150. doi:10.1136/bmjopen-2018-028150.

Chapter 1: Sleep 411

1. Garland SN, Rowe H, Repa LM, Fowler K, Zhou ES, Grandner MA. A decade's difference: 10-year change in insomnia symptom prevalence in Canada depends on sociodemographics and health status. *Sleep Health*. 2018 Apr;4(2):160-65. doi:10.1016/j.sleh.2018.01.003. Epub 2018 Feb 19. PMID: 29555129; PMCID: PMC6203592.
2. Moreno CRC, Conway SG, Assis M, Genta PR, Pachito DV, Tavares A Jr, Sguillar DA, Moreira G, Drager LF, Bacelar A. COVID-19 pandemic is associated with increased sleep disturbances and mental health symptoms but not help-seeking: a cross-sectional nation-wide study. *Sleep Science*. 2022 Jan–Mar; 15(1):1-7. doi:10.5935/1984-0063.20220027. PMID: 35662970; PMCID: PMC9153976.
3. Brinkman JE, Reddy V, Sharma S. Physiology of Sleep. 2023 Apr 3. *StatPearls*. Treasure Island (FL): StatPearls Publishing; April 2023. PMID: 29494118.
4. Brinkman JE, Reddy V, Sharma S. Physiology of Sleep. 2023 Apr 3. *StatPearls*. Treasure Island (FL): StatPearls Publishing; April 2023. PMID: 29494118.
5. Jung CM, Melanson EL, Frydendall EJ, Perreault L, Eckel RH, Wright KP. Energy expenditure during sleep, sleep deprivation and sleep following

sleep deprivation in adult humans. *J Physiol.* 2011 Jan 1;589(Pt 1):235-4. doi:10.1113/jphysiol.2010.197517. Epub 2010 Nov 8. PMID: 21059762; PMCID: PMC3039272.

6. Takahashi Y, Kipnis DM, Daughaday WH. Growth hormone secretion during sleep. *J Clin Invest.* 1968 Sep;47(9):2079–90. doi:10.1172/JCI105893. PMID: 5675428; PMCID: PMC297368.

7. Longo UG, Candela V, De Salvatore S, Piergentili I, Panattoni N, Casciani E, Faldetta A, Marchetti A, De Marinis MG, Denaro V. Arthroscopic Rotator Cuff Repair Improves Sleep Disturbance and Quality of Life: A Prospective Study. *Int J Environ Res Public Health.* 2021 Apr 6;18(7):3797. doi:10.3390/ijerph18073797. PMID: 33917277; PMCID: PMC8038746.

8. McAlpine CS, Kiss MG, Zuraikat FM, Cheek D, Schiroli G, Amatullah H, Huynh P, Bhatti MZ, Wong LP, Yates AG, Poller WC, Mindur JE, Chan CT, Janssen H, Downey J, Singh S, Sadreyev RI, Nahrendorf M, Jeffrey KL, Scadden DT, Naxerova K, St-Onge MP, Swirski FK. Sleep exerts lasting effects on hematopoietic stem cell function and diversity. *J Exp Med.* 2022 Nov 7; 219(11):e20220081. doi:10.1084/jem.20220081. Epub 2022 Sep 21. PMID: 36129517; PMCID: PMC9499822.

9. Seibt J, Frank MG. Primed to Sleep: The Dynamics of Synaptic Plasticity Across Brain States. *Front Syst Neurosci.* 2019 Feb 1;13:2. doi:10.3389/fnsys.2019.00002. PMID: 30774586; PMCID: PMC6367653.

10. Siegel JM. The neurotransmitters of sleep. *J Clin Psychiatry.* 2004;65(Suppl16):4-7. PMID: 15575797; PMCID: PMC8761080.

11. Lipinska G, Thomas KGF. The Interaction of REM Fragmentation and Night-Time Arousal Modulates Sleep-Dependent Emotional Memory Consolidation. *Front Psychol.* 2019 Aug 2;10:1766. doi:10.3389/fpsyg.2019.01766. PMID: 31428021; PMCID: PMC6688536.

12. Li W, Ma L, Yang G, Gan WB. REM sleep selectively prunes and maintains new synapses in development and learning. *Nat Neurosci.* 2017 Mar;20(3):427-37. doi:10.1038/nn.4479. Epub 2017 Jan 16. PMID: 28092659; PMCID: PMC5535798.

13. Walker M P, van der Helm E. Overnight therapy? The role of sleep in emotional brain processing. *Psychological Bulletin.* 2009;135(5):731-48. doi:10.1037/a0016570.

14. Ramireddy A, Chugh HS, Reinier K, Uy-Evanado A, Stecker EC, Jui J, Chugh SS. Sudden cardiac death during nighttime hours. *Heart Rhythm.* 2021 May;18(5):778-84. doi:10.1016/j.hrthm.2020.12.035. Epub 2021 Jan 20. PMID: 33482388; PMCID: PMC8096654.

15. Mackey J, Kleindorfer D, Sucharew H, Moomaw CJ, Kissela BM, Alwell K, Flaherty ML, Woo D, Khatri P, Adeoye O, Ferioli S, Khoury JC, Hornung

R, Broderick JP. Population-based study of wake-up strokes. *Neurology.* 2011 May 10;76(19):1662-67. doi:10.1212/WNL.0b013e318219fb30. PMID: 21555734; PMCID: PMC3100086.

16. Young T, Finn L, Peppard PE, Szklo-Coxe M, Austin D, Nieto FJ, Stubbs R, Hla KM. Sleep disordered breathing and mortality: eighteen-year follow-up of the Wisconsin sleep cohort. *Sleep.* 2008 Aug;31(8):1071-78. PMID: 18714778; PMCID: PMC2542952.

17. Milewski MD, Skaggs DL, Bishop GA, Pace JL, Ibrahim DA, Wren TA, Barzdukas A. Chronic lack of sleep is associated with increased sports injuries in adolescent athletes. *J Pediatr Orthop.* 2014 Mar;34(2):129-33. doi:10.1097/BPO.0000000000000151. PMID: 25028798.

18. Spiegel K, Tasali E, Penev P, Van Cauter E. Brief communication: Sleep curtailment in healthy young men is associated with decreased leptin levels, elevated ghrelin levels, and increased hunger and appetite. *Ann Intern Med.* 2004 Dec 7;141(11):846-50. doi:10.7326/0003-4819-141-11-200412070-00008. PMID: 15583226.

19. Saghir Z, Syeda JN, Muhammad AS, Balla Abdalla TH. The Amygdala, Sleep Debt, Sleep Deprivation, and the Emotion of Anger: A Possible Connection? *Cureus.* 2018 Jul 2;10(7):e2912. doi:10.7759/cureus.2912. PMID: 30186717; PMCID: PMC6122651.

20. Tomaso CC, Johnson AB, Nelson TD. The effect of sleep deprivation and restriction on mood, emotion, and emotion regulation: three meta-analyses in one. *Sleep.* 2021 Jun 11;44(6):zsaa289. doi:10.1093/sleep/zsaa289. PMID: 33367799; PMCID: PMC8193556.

21. Khan MA, Al-Jahdali H. The consequences of sleep deprivation on cognitive performance. *Neurosciences* (Riyadh). 2023 Apr;28(2):91-99. doi:10.17712/nsj.2023.2.20220108. PMID: 37045455; PMCID: PMC10155483.

22. LeBlanc ES, Smith NX, Nichols GA, et al. Insomnia is associated with an increased risk of type 2 diabetes in the clinical setting. *BMJ Open Diabetes Research and Care* 2018;6:e000604. doi:10.1136/bmjdrc-2018-000604.

23. Evbayekha EO, Aiwuyo HO, Dilibe A, Nriagu BN, Idowu AB, Eletta RY, Ohikhuai EE. Sleep Deprivation Is Associated With Increased Risk for Hypertensive Heart Disease: A Nationwide Population-Based Cohort Study. *Cureus.* 2022 Dec 27;14(12):e33005. doi:10.7759/cureus.33005. PMID: 36712752; PMCID: PMC9879308.

24. Everson CA, Bergmann BM, Rechtschaffen A. Sleep deprivation in the rat: III. Total sleep deprivation. *Sleep.* 1989 Feb;12(1):13-21. doi:10.1093/sleep/12.1.13. PMID: 2928622.

25. David Richter, Michael D Krämer, Nicole K Y Tang, Hawley E Montgomery-Downs, Sakari Lemola. Long-term effects of pregnancy and

childbirth on sleep satisfaction and duration of first-time and experienced mothers and fathers. *Sleep*, 42(4), April 2019, zsz015, doi:10.1093/sleep /zsz015.

26. Ross, J. J. (1965). Neurological findings after prolonged sleep deprivation. *Archives of Neurology*, 12(4), 399. doi:10.1001/archneur.1965.00460280069006.

27. Louca M, Short MA. The effect of one night's sleep deprivation on adolescent neurobehavioral performance. *Sleep*. 2014 Nov 1;37(11):1799-807. doi:10.5665/sleep.4174. PMID: 25364075; PMCID: PMC4196063.

28. Caccese JB, Iverson GL, Hunzinger KJ, Asken BM, Clugston JR, Cameron KL, Houston MN, Svoboda SJ, Jackson JC, McGinty GT, Estevez CA, Susmarski AJ, Enrique A, Bryk KN, Broglio SP, McAllister TW, McCrea M, Pasquina PF, Buckley TA; CARE Consortium Investigators. Factors Associated with Symptom Reporting in U.S. Service Academy Cadets and NCAA Student Athletes without Concussion: Findings from the CARE Consortium. *Sports Med*. 2021 May;51(5):1087-1105. doi:10.1007/s40279-020-01415-4. Epub 2021 Jan 11. PMID: 33428120.

29. National Highway Traffic Safety Administration. Drowsy Driving. https: //www.nhtsa.gov/risky-driving/drowsy-driving.

30. Schmid SM, Hallschmid M, Jauch-Chara K, Born J, Schultes B. A single night of sleep deprivation increases ghrelin levels and feelings of hunger in normal-weight healthy men. *J Sleep Res*. 2008 Sep;17(3):331-34. doi:10.1111 /j.1365-2869.2008.00662.x. Epub 2008 Jun 28. PMID: 18564298.

31. Waters F, Chiu V, Atkinson A, Blom JD. Severe Sleep Deprivation Causes Hallucinations and a Gradual Progression Toward Psychosis with Increasing Time Awake. *Front Psychiatry*. 2018 Jul 10;9:303. doi:10.3389/fpsyt.2018. 00303. PMID: 30042701; PMCID: PMC6048360.

32. Periasamy S, Hsu DZ, Fu YH, Liu MY. Sleep deprivation-induced multiorgan injury: role of oxidative stress and inflammation. *EXCLI J*. 2015 May 18;14:672-83. doi:10.17179/excli2015-245. PMID: 26648820; PMCID: PMC4669910.

Chapter 2: Sleep Assessment Tools

1. Hirshkowitz M, Whiton K, Albert SM, Alessi C, Bruni O, DonCarlos L, Hazen N, Herman J, Katz ES, Kheirandish-Gozal L, Neubauer DN, O'Donnell AE, Ohayon M, Peever J, Rawding R, Sachdeva RC, Setters B, Vitiello MV, Ware JC, Adams Hillard PJ. National Sleep Foundation's sleep time duration recommendations: methodology and results summary. *Sleep Health*. 2015 Mar;1(1):40-43. doi:10.1016/j.sleh.2014.12.010. Epub 2015 Jan 8. PMID: 29073412.

2. Barbato G. REM Sleep: An Unknown Indicator of Sleep Quality. *Int J Environ Res Public Health*. 2021 Dec 9;18(24):12976. doi:10.3390/ijerph182412976.

PMID: 34948586; PMCID: PMC8702162.

3. Buysse DJ, Reynolds CF 3rd, Monk TH, Berman SR, Kupfer DJ. The Pittsburgh Sleep Quality Index: a new instrument for psychiatric practice and research. *Psychiatry Res.* 1989 May;28(2):193-213. doi:10.1016/0165-1781(89)90047-4. PMID: 2748771.

4. Trotti LM. Waking up is the hardest thing I do all day: Sleep inertia and sleep drunkenness. *Sleep Med Rev.* 2017 Oct;35:76-84. doi:10.1016/j.smrv.2016.08.005. Epub 2016 Sep 4. PMID: 27692973; PMCID: PMC5337178.

5. Lee JM, Byun W, Keill A, Dinkel D, Seo Y. Comparison of Wearable Trackers' Ability to Estimate Sleep. *Int J Environ Res Public Health.* 2018 Jun 15;15(6):1265. doi:10.3390/ijerph15061265. PMID: 29914050; PMCID: PMC6025478.

Chapter 3: Troubleshooting Sleep

1. Cohen S, Doyle WJ, Alper CM, Janicki-Deverts D, Turner RB. Sleep habits and susceptibility to the common cold. *Arch Intern Med.* 2009 Jan 12;169(1):62-67. doi:10.1001/archinternmed.2008.505. PMID: 19139325; PMCID: PMC2629403.

2. Irwin M, Mascovich A, Gillin JC, Willoughby R, Pike J, Smith TL. Partial sleep deprivation reduces natural killer cell activity in humans. *Psychosom Med.* 1994 Nov-Dec;56(6):493-98. doi:10.1097/00006842-199411000-00004. PMID: 7871104.

3. Shan Z, Ma H, Xie M, et al. Sleep duration and risk of type 2 diabetes: A meta-analysis of prospective studies. *Diabetes Care,* 2015;38(3):529-37. doi:10.2337/dc14-2073.

4. Cappuccio FP, Cooper D, D'Elia L, Strazzullo P, Miller MA. Sleep duration predicts cardiovascular outcomes: A systematic review and meta-analysis of prospective studies. *European Heart Journal.* 2011;32(12):1484-92. doi:10.1093/eurheartj/ehr007.

5. Dzierzewski JM, Donovan EK, Kay DB, Sannes TS, Bradbrook KE. Sleep Inconsistency and Markers of Inflammation. *Front Neurol.* 2020 Sep 16;11:1042. doi:10.3389/fneur.2020.01042. PMID: 33041983; PMCID: PMC7525126.

6. Bak LK, Walls AB, Schousboe A, Waagepetersen HS. Astrocytic glycogen metabolism in the healthy and diseased brain. *J Biol Chem.* 2018 May 11;293(19):7108-16. doi:10.1074/jbc.R117.803239. Epub 2018 Mar 23. PMID: 29572349; PMCID: PMC5950001.

7. Herring MP, Monroe DC, Kline CE, O'Connor PJ, MacDonncha C. Sleep quality moderates the association between physical activity frequency and feelings of energy and fatigue in adolescents. *Eur Child Adolesc Psychiatry.* 2018 Nov;27(11):1425-32. doi:10.1007/s00787-018-1134-z. Epub 2018 Mar

5. PMID: 29508054; PMCID: PMC6410735.

8. Bailey BW, Allen MD, LeCheminant JD, Tucker LA, Errico WK, Christensen WF, Hill MD. Objectively measured sleep patterns in young adult women and the relationship to adiposity. *Am J Health Promot.* 2014 Sep;29(1):46-54. doi:10.4278/ajhp.121012-QUAN-500. Epub 2013 Nov 7. PMID: 24200246.

9. Hasler G, Buysse DJ, Klaghofer R, Gamma A, Ajdacic V, Eich D, Rössler W, Angst J. The association between short sleep duration and obesity in young adults: a 13-year prospective study. *Sleep.* 2004 Jun 15;27(4):661-66. doi:10.1093/sleep/27.4.661. PMID: 15283000.

10. Spiegel K, Tasali E, Penev P, Van Cauter E. Brief communication: Sleep curtailment in healthy young men is associated with decreased leptin levels, elevated ghrelin levels, and increased hunger and appetite. *Ann Intern Med.* 2004 Dec 7;141(11):846-50. doi:10.7326/0003-4819-141-11-200412070-00008. PMID: 15583226.

11. National Heart, Lung, and Blood Institute. *Your Guide to Healthy Sleep.* 2011 Aug, https://www.nhlbi.nih.gov/resources/your-guide-healthy-sleep.

12. Division of Sleep Medicine at Harvard Medical School. Sleep and disease risk. *Why Sleep Matters: Consequences of Sleep Deficiency.* 2021 Oct. https://sleep.hms.harvard.edu/education-training/public-education/sleep-and-health-education-program/sleep-health-education-45.

13. Li SH, Corkish B, Richardson C, Christensen H, Werner-Seidler A. The role of rumination in the relationship between symptoms of insomnia and depression in adolescents. *J Sleep Res.* 2023 May 17:e13932. doi:10.1111/jsr.13932. Epub ahead of print. PMID: 37198139.

14. Vandekerckhove M, Wang YL. Emotion, emotion regulation and sleep: An intimate relationship. *AIMS Neurosci.* 2017 Dec 1;5(1):1-17. doi:10.3934/Neuroscience.2018.1.1. PMID: 32341948; PMCID: PMC7181893.

15. Yap Y, Slavish DC, Taylor DJ, Bei B, Wiley JF. Bi-directional relations between stress and self-reported and actigraphy-assessed sleep: a daily intensive longitudinal study. *Sleep.* 2020 Mar 12;43(3):zsz250. doi:10.1093/sleep/zsz250. PMID: 31608395; PMCID: PMC7066487.

16. Leary EB, Watson KT, Ancoli-Israel S, Redline S, Yaffe K, Ravelo LA, Peppard PE, Zou J, Goodman SN, Mignot E, Stone KL. Association of Rapid Eye Movement Sleep with Mortality in Middle-aged and Older Adults. *JAMA Neurol.* 2020 Oct 1;77(10):1241-51. doi:10.1001/jamaneurol.2020.2108. Erratum in: *JAMA Neurol.* 2020 Oct 1;77(10):1322. PMID: 32628261; PMCID: PMC7550971.

17. Mazzoccoli G, Sothern R, Francavilla M, De Petris M, Giuliani F. Comparison of whole body circadian phase evaluated from melatonin and

cortisol secretion profiles in healthy humans. *Biomedicine & Aging Pathology.* 2011;1(2). doi:10.1016/j.biomag.2011.06.006.

18. Jike M, Itani O, Watanabe N, Buysse DJ, Kaneita Y. Long sleep duration and health outcomes: A systematic review, meta-analysis and meta-regression. *Sleep Med Rev.* 2018 Jun;39:25-36. doi:10.1016/j.smrv.2017.06.011. Epub 2017 Jul 5. PMID: 28890167.

19. Nutt D, Wilson S, Paterson L. Sleep disorders as core symptoms of depression. *Dialogues Clin Neurosci.* 2008;10(3):329-36. doi:10.31887/DCNS.2008. 10.3/dnutt. PMID: 18979946; PMCID: PMC3181883.

20. Geoffroy PA, Hoertel N, Etain B, Bellivier F, Delorme R, Limosin F, Peyre H. Insomnia and hypersomnia in major depressive episode: Prevalence, sociodemographic characteristics and psychiatric comorbidity in a population-based study. *J Affect Disord.* 2018 Jan 15;226:132-41. doi:10.1016/j .jad.2017.09.032. Epub 2017 Sep 25. PMID: 28972930.

21. Roehrs T, Roth T. Sleep, sleepiness, and alcohol use. *Alcohol Res Health.* 2001;25(2):101-09. PMID: 11584549; PMCID: PMC6707127.

22. Wetter DW, Young TB. The relation between cigarette smoking and sleep disturbance. *Prev Med.* 1994 May;23(3):328-34. doi:10.1006/pmed.1994. 1046. PMID: 8078854.

23. Vaillancourt R, Gallagher S, Cameron JD, Dhalla R. Cannabis use in patients with insomnia and sleep disorders: Retrospective chart review. *Can Pharm J* (Ott). 2022 Apr 15;155(3):175-80. doi:10.1177/17151635221089617. PMID: 35519083; PMCID: PMC9067069.

24. Grotenhermen F. Pharmacokinetics and pharmacodynamics of cannabinoids. *Clin Pharmacokinet.* 2003;42(4):327-60. doi:10.2165/00003088-200342040-00003. PMID: 12648025.

25. Betts TA, Alford C. Beta-blockers and sleep: a controlled trial. *Eur J Clin Pharmacol.* 1985;28 Suppl:65-68. doi:10.1007/BF00543712. PMID: 2865152.

26. Yang CC, Chien WC, Chung CH, Lai CY, Tzeng NS. The Usage of Histamine Type 1 Receptor Antagonist and Risk of Dementia in the Elderly: A Nationwide Cohort Study. *Front Aging Neurosci.* 2022 Mar 18;14:811494. doi:10.3389/fnagi.2022.811494. PMID: 35370616; PMCID: PMC8972197.

27. Morin CM, Jarrin DC. Epidemiology of Insomnia: Prevalence, Course, Risk Factors, and Public Health Burden. *Sleep Med Clin.* 2022 Jun;17(2):173-91. doi:10.1016/j.jsmc.2022.03.003. Epub 2022 Apr 23. PMID: 35659072.

Chapter 4: Sleep for the Win

1. Besedovsky L, Lange T, Born J. Sleep and immune function. *Pflugers Arch.* 2012 Jan;463(1):121-37. doi:10.1007/s00424-011-1044-0. Epub 2011 Nov 10. PMID: 22071480; PMCID: PMC3256323.

2. Schmitz NCM, van der Werf YD, Lammers-van der Holst HM. The Importance of Sleep and Circadian Rhythms for Vaccination Success and Susceptibility to Viral Infections. *Clocks Sleep.* 2022 Feb 16;4(1):66-79. doi:10.3390/clockssleep4010008. PMID: 35225954; PMCID: PMC8884008.

3. McAlpine CS, Kiss MG, Zuraikat FM, et al. Sleep exerts lasting effects on hematopoietic stem cell function and diversity. *J Exp Med.* 2022 Nov 7;219(11):e20220081. doi:10.1084/jem.20220081. Epub 2022 Sep 21. PMID: 36129517; PMCID: PMC9499822.

4. Kline CE. The bidirectional relationship between exercise and sleep: Implications for exercise adherence and sleep improvement. *Am J Lifestyle Med.* 2014 Nov-Dec;8(6):375-79. doi:10.1177/1559827614544437. PMID: 25729341; PMCID: PMC4341978.

5. Nedeltcheva AV, Kilkus JM, Imperial J, Schoeller DA, Penev PD. Insufficient sleep undermines dietary efforts to reduce adiposity. *Ann Intern Med.* 2010 Oct 5;153(7):435-41. doi:10.7326/0003-4819-153-7-201010050-00006. PMID: 20921542; PMCID: PMC2951287.

6. Frank S, Gonzalez K, Lee-Ang L, Young MC, Tamez M, Mattei J. Diet and Sleep Physiology: Public Health and Clinical Implications. *Front Neurol.* 2017 Aug 11;8:393. doi:10.3389/fneur.2017.00393. PMID: 28848491; PMCID: PMC5554513.

7. Cai DJ, Mednick SA, Harrison EM, Kanady JC, Mednick SC. REM, not incubation, improves creativity by priming associative networks. *Proc Natl Acad Sci.* 2009 Jun 23;106(25):10130-34. doi:10.1073/pnas.0900271106. Epub 2009 Jun 8. PMID: 19506253; PMCID: PMC2700890.

8. Horowitz AH, Esfahany K, Gálvez TV, Maes P, Stickgold R. Targeted dream incubation at sleep onset increases post-sleep creative performance. *Sci Rep.* 2023 May 15;13(1):7319. doi:10.1038/s41598-023-31361-w. PMID: 37188795; PMCID: PMC10185495.

9. Windred DP, Burns AC, Lane JM, Saxena R, Rutter MK, Cain SW, Phillips AJK. Sleep regularity is a stronger predictor of mortality risk than sleep duration: A prospective cohort study. *Sleep.* 2023 Sep 21:zsad253. doi:10.1093/sleep/zsad253. Epub ahead of print. PMID: 37738616.

10. Briken P, Matthiesen S, Pietras L, Wiessner C, Klein V, Reed GM, Dekker A. Estimating the Prevalence of Sexual Dysfunction Using the New ICD-11 Guidelines. *Dtsch Arztebl Int.* 2020 Sep 25;117(39):653-658. doi:10.3238/arztebl.2020.0653. PMID: 33357346; PMCID: PMC7829447.

11. Kalmbach DA, Arnedt JT, Pillai V, Ciesla JA. The impact of sleep on female sexual response and behavior: a pilot study. *J Sex Med.* 2015 May;12(5):1221-32. doi:10.1111/jsm.12858. Epub 2015 Mar 16. PMID: 25772315.

12. Wilson SJ, Jaremka LM, Fagundes CP, Andridge R, Peng J, Malarkey WB, Habash D, Belury MA, Kiecolt-Glaser JK. Shortened sleep fuels

inflammatory responses to marital conflict: Emotion regulation matters. *Psychoneuroendocrinology*. 2017 May;79:74-83. doi:10.1016/j.psyneuen.2017 .02.015. Epub 2017 Feb 16. PMID: 28262602; PMCID: PMC5419294.

13. Chen KF, Liang SJ, Lin CL, Liao WC, Kao CH. Sleep disorders increase risk of subsequent erectile dysfunction in individuals without sleep apnea: a nationwide population-base cohort study. *Sleep Med*. 2016 Jan;17:64-68. doi:10.1016/j.sleep.2015.05.018. Epub 2015 Jun 29. PMID: 26847976.

14. Wilson SJ, Jaremka LM, Fagundes CP, Andridge R, Peng J, Malarkey WB, Habash D, Belury MA, Kiecolt-Glaser JK. Shortened sleep fuels inflammatory responses to marital conflict: Emotion regulation matters. *Psychoneuroendocrinology*. 2017 May;79:74-83. doi:10.1016/j.psyneuen.2017.02.015. Epub 2017 Feb 16. PMID: 28262602; PMCID: PMC5419294.

15. Backhaus J, Junghanns K, Hohagen F. Sleep disturbances are correlated with decreased morning awakening salivary cortisol. *Psychoneuroendocrinology*. 2004 Oct;29(9):1184-91. doi:10.1016/j.psyneuen.2004.01.010. PMID: 15219642.

16. Wehrens SMT, Christou S, Isherwood C, Middleton B, Gibbs MA, Archer SN, Skene DJ, Johnston JD. Meal Timing Regulates the Human Circadian System. *Curr Biol*. 2017 Jun 19;27(12):1768-75.e3. doi:10.1016/j.cub.2017.04 .059. Epub 2017 Jun 1. PMID: 28578930; PMCID: PMC5483233.

17. Costello HM, Johnston JG, Juffre A, Crislip GR, Gumz ML. Circadian clocks of the kidney: function, mechanism, and regulation. *Physiol Rev*. 2022 Oct 1;102(4):1669-1701. doi:10.1152/physrev.00045.2021. Epub 2022 May 16. PMID: 35575250; PMCID: PMC9273266.

18. Saidi O, Peyrel P, Del Sordo G, Gabriel B, Maso F, Doré É, Duché P. Is it wiser to train in the afternoon or the early evening to sleep better? The role of chronotype in young adolescent athletes. *Sleep*. 2023 Jul 11;46(7):zsad099. doi:10.1093/sleep/zsad099. PMID: 37018755.

19. Riedy SM, Smith MG, Rocha S, Basner M. Noise as a sleep aid: A systematic review. *Sleep Med Rev*. 2021 Feb;55:101385. doi:10.1016/j.smrv.2020. 101385. Epub 2020 Sep 9. PMID: 33007706.

20. Raj A, Ruder M, Rus HM, Gahan L, O'Mullane B, Danoff-Burg S, Raymann R. 1214 Higher Bedroom Temperature Associated With Poorer Sleep: Data From Over 3.75 Million Nights. *Sleep* 43 Supplement 1, 2020 April;A464. doi:10.1093/sleep/zsaa056.1208.

21. United States Environmental Protection Agency, "Care for Your Air: A Guide to Indoor Air Quality." https://www.epa.gov/indoor-air-quality -iaq/care-your-air-guide-indoor-air-quality.

22. Faraut B, Nakib S, Drogou C, Elbaz M, Sauvet F, De Bandt JP, Léger D. Napping reverses the salivary interleukin-6 and urinary norepinephrine changes induced by sleep restriction. *J Clin Endocrinol Metab*. 2015

Mar;100(3):E416-26. doi:10.1210/jc.2014-2566. Epub 2015 Feb 10. PMID: 25668196.

23. Souabni M, Hammouda O, Romdhani M, Trabelsi K, Ammar A, Driss T. Benefits of Daytime Napping Opportunity on Physical and Cognitive Performances in Physically Active Participants: A Systematic Review. *Sports Med.* 2021 Oct;51(10):2115-46. doi:10.1007/s40279-021-01482-1. Epub 2021 May 27. PMID: 34043185.

24. Yang Y, Liu W, Ji X, Ma C, Wang X, Li K, Li J. Extended afternoon naps are associated with hypertension in women but not in men. *Heart Lung.* 2020 Jan-Feb;49(1):2-9. doi:10.1016/j.hrtlng.2019.09.002. Epub 2019 Sep 11. PMID: 31521340; PMCID: PMC6961342.

25. Lam KB, Jiang CQ, Thomas GN, Arora T, Zhang WS, Taheri S, Adab P, Lam TH, Cheng KK. Napping is associated with increased risk of type 2 diabetes: the Guangzhou Biobank Cohort Study. *Sleep.* 2010 Mar;33(3):402-07. doi:10.1093/sleep/33.3.402. PMID: 20337199; PMCID: PMC2831435.

26. Zhang H, Zhang L, Chen C, Zhong X. Association between daytime napping and cognitive impairment among Chinese older population: a cross-sectional study. *Environ Health Prev Med.* 2023;28:72. doi:10.1265/ehpm .23-00031. PMID: 37989282; PMCID: PMC10685077.

27. Meaklim H, Le F, Drummond SPA, Bains SK, Varma P, Junge MF, Jackson ML. Insomnia is more likely to persist than remit after a time of stress and uncertainty: A longitudinal cohort study examining trajectories and predictors of insomnia symptoms. *Sleep.* 2024 Feb 3:zsae028. doi:10.1093/sleep /zsae028. Epub ahead of print. PMID: 38308584.

Chapter 5: Drink 411

1. Bouby N, Fernandes S. Mild dehydration, vasopressin and the kidney: animal and human studies. *Eur J Clin Nutr.* 2003 Dec;57 Suppl 2:S39-46. doi:10.1038/sj.ejcn.1601900. PMID: 14681712.

2. Brooks CJ, Gortmaker SL, Long MW, Cradock AL, Kenney EL. Racial/ Ethnic and Socioeconomic Disparities in Hydration Status Among US Adults and the Role of Tap Water and Other Beverage Intake. *Am J Public Health.* 2017 Sep;107(9):1387-94. doi:10.2105/AJPH.2017.303923. Epub 2017 Jul 20. PMID: 28727528; PMCID: PMC5551608.

3. Taylor K, Jones EB. Adult Dehydration. StatPearls. Treasure Island (FL): *StatPearls* Publishing; 2022 Oct. https://www.ncbi.nlm.nih.gov/books /NBK555956.

4. Augustine V, Ebisu H, Zhao Y, Lee S, Ho B, Mizuno GO, Tian L, Oka Y. Temporally and Spatially Distinct Thirst Satiation Signals. *Neuron.* 2019 Jul 17;103(2):242-49.e4. doi:10.1016/j.neuron.2019.04.039. Epub 2019 May 29. PMID: 31153646; PMCID: PMC7335596.

5. Augustine V, Gokce S, Lee S, et al. Hierarchical neural architecture underlying thirst regulation. *Nature* 2018;555, 204–09. https://doi.org/10.1038/nature25488.

6. Millard-Stafford M, Wendland DM, O'Dea NK, Norman TL. Thirst and hydration status in everyday life. *Nutr Rev.* 2012 Nov;70 Suppl 2:S147-51.

Chapter 6: Drink Assessment Tools

1. Goehring MT, Farran J, Ingles-Laughlin C, Benedista-Seelman S, Williams B. Measures of Skin Turgor in Humans: A Systematic Review of the Literature. *Wound Manag Prev.* 2022 Apr;68(4):14-24. doi:10.25270/wmp.2022.4.1424. PMID: 35544778.

2. Çiftçi B, Yıldız GN, Avşar G, Köse S, Aydın E, Doğan S, Çelik Ş. Development of the Thirst Discomfort Scale: A Validity and Reliability Study. *Am J Crit Care.* 2023 May 1;32(3):176-83. doi:10.4037/ajcc2023954. PMID: 37121897.

3. Wyman JF, Cain CH, Epperson CN, Fitzgerald CM, Gahagan S, Newman DK, Rudser K, Smith AL, Vaughan CP, Sutcliffe S. Prevention of Lower Urinary Tract Symptoms (PLUS) Research Consortium. Urination Frequency Ranges in Healthy Women. *Nurs Res.* 2022 Sep-Oct;71(5):341-52. doi:10.1097/NNR.0000000000000595. Epub 2022 Mar 22. PMID: 35319538; PMCID: PMC9420750.

4. Eggleton MG. The diuretic action of alcohol in man. *J Physiol.* 1942 Aug 18;101(2):172-91. doi:10.1113/jphysiol.1942.sp003973. PMID: 16991552; PMCID: PMC1393383.

5. Maughan R, Griffin J. Caffeine ingestion and fluid balance: A review. *Journal of human nutrition and dietetics: the official journal of the British Dietetic Association.* 2003;16. 411-20. doi:10.1046/j.1365-277X.2003.00477.x.

6. The National Academy of Sciences. *Dietary References Intakes for Water, Potassium, Sodium, Chloride, and Sulfate.* National Academies Press, 2005. https://www.nap.edu/read/10925/chapter/6#102.

7. Yang P, Pham J, Choo J, Hu D. Duration of urination does not change with body size. *Proceedings of the National Academy of Sciences.* 2014 Aug 19;111(33):11932-37. doi:10.1073/pnas.1402289111.

Chapter 7: Troubleshooting Drink

1. Taylor K, Jones EB. Adult Dehydration. StatPearls. Treasure Island (FL): StatPearls Publishing; 2022 Oct. https://www.ncbi.nlm.nih.gov/books/NBK555956.

2. Ayotte D Jr, Corcoran MP. Individualized hydration plans improve performance outcomes for collegiate athletes engaging in in-season training. *J Int Soc Sports Nutr.* 2018 Jun 4;15(1):27. doi:10.1186/s12970-018-0230-2.

PMID: 29866199; PMCID: PMC5987390.

3. Barley OR, Chapman DW, Blazevich AJ, Abbiss CR. Acute Dehydration Impairs Endurance Without Modulating Neuromuscular Function. *Front Physiol.* 2018 Nov 2;9:1562. doi:10.3389/fphys.2018.01562. PMID: 30450056; PMCID: PMC6224374.

4. Ganio MS, Armstrong LE, Casa DJ, McDermott BP, Lee EC, Yamamoto LM, Marzano S, Lopez RM, Jimenez L, Le Bellego L, Chevillotte E, Lieberman HR. Mild dehydration impairs cognitive performance and mood of men. *Br J Nutr.* 2011 Nov;106(10):1535-43. doi:10.1017/S0007114511002005. Epub 2011 Jun 7. PMID: 21736786.

5. Stachenfeld NS, Leone CA, Mitchell ES, Freese E, Harkness L. Water intake reverses dehydration associated impaired executive function in healthy young women. *Physiol Behav.* 2018 Mar 1;185:103-11. doi:10.1016/j.physbeh.2017.12.028. Epub 2017 Dec 23. PMID: 29277553.

6. Zhang N, Du SM, Zhang JF, Ma GS. Effects of Dehydration and Rehydration on Cognitive Performance and Mood among Male College Students in Cangzhou, China: A Self-Controlled Trial. *Int J Environ Res Public Health.* 2019 May 29;16(11):1891. doi:10.3390/ijerph16111891. PMID: 31146326; PMCID: PMC6603652.

7. Spigt M, Weerkamp N, Troost J, van Schayck CP, Knottnerus JA. A randomized trial on the effects of regular water intake in patients with recurrent headaches. *Fam Pract.* 2012 Aug;29(4):370-75. doi:10.1093/fampra/cmr112. Epub 2011 Nov 23. PMID: 22113647.

8. Hamrick I, Norton D, Birstler J, Chen G, Cruz L, Hanrahan L. Association Between Dehydration and Falls. *Mayo Clin Proc Innov Qual Outcomes.* 2020 Jun 5;4(3):259-65. doi:10.1016/j.mayocpiqo.2020.01.003. PMID: 32542217; PMCID: PMC7283563.

9. Schuster BG, Kosar L, Kamrul R. Constipation in older adults: stepwise approach to keep things moving. *Can Fam Physician.* 2015 Feb;61(2):152-58. PMID: 25676646; PMCID: PMC4325863.

10. Arnaoutis G, Kavouras SA, Stratakis N, et al. The effect of hypohydration on endothelial function in young healthy adults. *Eur J Nutr* 2017;56:1211-17. doi:10.1007/s00394-016-1170-8.

11. Tannenbaum E. Brooke Shields Recently Experienced a "Full-Blown" Seizure—and Bradley Cooper Came Running. *Glamour.* November 1, 2023.

12. Rosinger AY, Chang A-M, Buxton OM, Li J, Wu S, Gao X, Short sleep duration is associated with inadequate hydration: cross-cultural evidence from US and Chinese adults. *Sleep.* 2019 Feb;42(2), doi:10.1093/sleep/zsy210.

13. Retallick-Brown H, Blampied N, Rucklidge JJ. A Pilot Randomized Treatment-Controlled Trial Comparing Vitamin B6 with Broad-Spectrum Micronutrients for Premenstrual Syndrome. *J Altern Complement Med.*

2020 Feb;26(2):88-97. doi:10.1089/acm.2019.0305. Epub 2020 Jan 10. PMID: 31928364.

14. Maughan RJ, Griffin J. Caffeine ingestion and fluid balance: a review. *J Hum Nutr Diet.* 2003 Dec;16(6):411-20. doi:10.1046/j.1365-277x.2003.00477.x. PMID: 19774754.

15. Wei J, Zhao M, Meng K, Xia G, Pan Y, Li C, Zhang W. The Diuretic Effects of Coconut Water by Suppressing Aquaporin and Renin-Angiotensin-Aldosterone System in Saline-Loaded Rats. *Front Nutr.* 2022 Jun 23;9:930506. doi:10.3389/fnut.2022.930506. PMID: 35811978; PMCID: PMC9262403.

16. El-Tawil AM. Colorectal cancers and chlorinated water. *World J Gastrointest Oncol.* 2016 Apr 15;8(4):402-09. doi:10.4251/wjgo.v8.i4.402. PMID: 27096035; PMCID: PMC4824718.

17. University of Hawaii at Manoa. Petroleum, chlorine mix could yield harmful byproducts. *ScienceDaily.* 2024 May 14. https://www.sciencedaily.com/releases/2024/05/240514183448.htm.

18. Gonsioroski A, Mourikes VE, Flaws JA. Endocrine Disruptors in Water and Their Effects on the Reproductive System. *Int J Mol Sci.* 2020 Mar 12;21(6):1929. doi:10.3390/ijms21061929. PMID: 32178293; PMCID: PMC7139484.

19. Qian N, Gao X, Lang X, Deng H, Bratu TM, Chen Q, Stapleton P, Yan B, Min W. Rapid single-particle chemical imaging of nanoplastics by SRS microscopy. *Proc Natl Acad Sci.* 2024 Jan 16;121(3):e2300582121. doi:10.1073/pnas.2300582121. Epub 2024 Jan 8. PMID: 38190543; PMCID: PMC10801917.

Chapter 8: Drink for the Win

1. Bergstrom K, Shan X, Casero D, Batushansky A, Lagishetty V, Jacobs JP, Hoover C, Kondo Y, Shao B, Gao L, Zandberg W, Noyovitz B, McDaniel JM, Gibson DL, Pakpour S, Kazemian N, McGee S, Houchen CW, Rao CV, Griffin TM, Sonnenburg JL, McEver RP, Braun J, Xia L. Proximal colon-derived O-glycosylated mucus encapsulates and modulates the microbiota. *Science.* 2020 Oct 23;370(6515):467-72. doi:10.1126/science.aay7367. PMID: 33093110; PMCID: PMC8132455

2. Hansson GC. Role of mucus layers in gut infection and inflammation. *Curr Opin Microbiol.* 2012 Feb;15(1):57-62. doi:10.1016/j.mib.2011.11.002. Epub 2011 Dec 14. PMID: 22177113; PMCID: PMC3716454

3. Suriano F, Nyström EEL, Sergi D, Gustafsson JK. Diet, microbiota, and the mucus layer: The guardians of our health. *Front Immunol.* 2022 Sep 13;13:953196. doi:10.3389/fimmu.2022.953196. PMID: 36177011; PMCID: PMC9513540.

4. Bothe G, Coh A, Auinger A. Efficacy and safety of a natural mineral water

rich in magnesium and sulphate for bowel function: a double-blind, randomized, placebo-controlled study. *Eur J Nutr.* 2017 Mar;56(2):491-99. doi:10.1007/s00394-015-1094-8. Epub 2015 Nov 18. PMID: 26582579; PMCID: PMC5334415.

5. Zhou HL, Wei MH, Cui Y, Di DS, Song WJ, Zhang RY, Liu JA, Wang Q. Association Between Water Intake and Mortality Risk-Evidence From a National Prospective Study. *Front Nutr.* 2022 Apr 12;9:822119. doi:10.3389/fnut.2022.822119. PMID: 35495952; PMCID: PMC9039539.

6. Dmitrieva NI, Gagarin A, Liu D, Wu CO, Boehm M. Middle-age high normal serum sodium as a risk factor for accelerated biological aging, chronic diseases, and premature mortality. *EBioMedicine.* 2023 Jan;87:104404. doi:10.1016/j.ebiom.2022.104404. Epub 2023 Jan 2. PMID: 36599719; PMCID: PMC9873684.

7. Dmitrieva NI, Gagarin A, Liu D, Wu CO, Boehm M. Middle-age high normal serum sodium as a risk factor for accelerated biological aging, chronic diseases, and premature mortality. *EBioMedicine.* 2023 Jan;87:104404. doi:10.1016/j.ebiom.2022.104404. Epub 2023 Jan 2. PMID: 36599719; PMCID: PMC9873684.

8. Davy BM, Dennis EA, Dengo AL, Wilson KL, Davy KP. Water consumption reduces energy intake at a breakfast meal in obese older adults. *J Am Diet Assoc.* 2008 Jul;108(7):1236-39. doi:10.1016/j.jada.2008.04.013. PMID: 18589036; PMCID: PMC2743119.

9. Vij VA, Joshi AS. Effect of "water induced thermogenesis" on body weight, body mass index and body composition of overweight subjects. *J Clin Diagn Res.* 2013 Sep;7(9):1894-96. doi:10.7860/JCDR/2013/5862.3344. Epub 2013 Sep 10. PMID: 24179891; PMCID: PMC3809630.

10. Boschmann M, Steiniger J, Hille U, Tank J, Adams F, Sharma AM, Klaus S, Luft FC, Jordan J. Water-induced thermogenesis. *J Clin Endocrinol Metab.* 2003 Dec;88(12):6015-19. doi:10.1210/jc.2003-030780. PMID: 14671205.

11. Paik IY, Jeong MH, Jin HE, Kim YI, Suh AR, Cho SY, Roh HT, Jin CH, Suh SH. Fluid replacement following dehydration reduces oxidative stress during recovery. *Biochem Biophys Res Commun.* 2009 May 22;383(1):103-07. doi:10.1016/j.bbrc.2009.03.135. Epub 2009 Apr 1. PMID: 19344695.

12. Pawson C, Gardner M, Doherty S, Martin L, Soares R, Edmonds CJ. Drink availability is associated with enhanced examination performance in adults. *Psychology Teaching Review.* 2013;19(1):57-66.

13. Arca KN, Halker Singh RB. Dehydration and Headache. *Curr Pain Headache Rep.* 2021 Jul 15;25(8):56. doi:10.1007/s11916-021-00966-z. PMID: 34268642; PMCID: PMC8280611.

14. Sawka MN, Cheuvront SN, Carter R. Human Water Needs, *Nutrition*

Reviews. 2005 June:63(Suppl 1): S30–S39. doi:10.1111/j.1753-4887.2005. tb00152.x

15. Yamada Y, Zhang X, et al. Variation in human water turnover associated with environmental and lifestyle factors. *Science.* 2022 Nov 25;378(6622):909915. doi:10.1126/science.abm8668. Epub 2022 Nov 24. PMID: 36423296; PMCID: PMC9764345.

16. Papies E, Rodger A, Almudena Claassen M, Lomann M. Recent Findings on the Psychology of Hydration Habits. *Ann Nutr Metab.* 28 December 2021;77(Suppl. 4):15–16. doi:10.1159/000520781.

17. Hooper L, Abdelhamid A, Attreed NJ, Campbell WW, Channell AM, et al. Clinical symptoms, signs and tests for identification of impending and current water-loss dehydration in older people. *Cochrane Database Syst Rev.* 2015 Apr 30;(4):CD009647.

18. US Food and Drug Administration. *Food Facts: Sodium in Your Diet.* 2021 June. https://www.fda.gov/food/nutrition-education-resources-materials /sodium-your-diet.

19. Choi D, Cho J, Koo J, Kim T. Effects of Electrolyte Supplements on Body Water Homeostasis and Exercise Performance during Exhaustive Exercise. *Applied Sciences.* 2021;11. 9093. doi:10.3390/app11199093.

20. Nieman DC, Gillitt ND, Sha W, Esposito D, Ramamoorthy S. Metabolic recovery from heavy exertion following banana compared to sugar beverage or water only ingestion: A randomized, crossover trial. *PLoS One.* 2018 Mar 22;13(3):e0194843. doi:10.1371/journal.pone.0194843. PMID: 29566095; PMCID: PMC5864065.

21. Crous-Bou M, Molinuevo JL, Sala-Vila A. Plant-Rich Dietary Patterns, Plant Foods and Nutrients, and Telomere Length. *Adv Nutr.* 2019 Nov 1;10(Suppl_4):S296-S303. doi:10.1093/advances/nmz026. PMID: 31728493; PMCID: PMC6855941.

22. Popkin BM, D'Anci KE, Rosenberg IH. Water, hydration, and health. *Nutr Rev.* 2010 Aug;68(8):439-58. doi:10.1111/j.1753-4887.2010.00304.x. PMID: 20646222; PMCID: PMC2908954.

23. US Food and Drug Administration. CFR—Code of Federal Regulations, Title 21, Part 165, Beverages. 2023 Dec 22. https://www.accessdata.fda.gov /scripts/cdrh/cfdocs/cfcfr/CFRSearch.cfm?CFRPart=165.

24. Song G, Li M, Sang H, Zhang L, Li X, Yao S, Yu Y, Zong C, Xue Y, Qin S. Hydrogen-rich water decreases serum LDL-cholesterol levels and improves HDL function in patients with potential metabolic syndrome. *J Lipid Res.* 2013 Jul;54(7):1884-93. doi:10.1194/jlr.M036640. Epub 2013 Apr 22. PMID: 23610159; PMCID: PMC3679390.

25. Mizuno K, Sasaki AT, Ebisu K, Tajima K, Kajimoto O, Nojima J,

Kuratsune H, Hori H, Watanabe Y. Hydrogen-rich water for improvements of mood, anxiety, and autonomic nerve function in daily life. *Med Gas Res.* 2018 Jan 22;7(4):247-55. doi:10.4103/2045-9912.222448. PMID: 29497485; PMCID: PMC5806445.

26. Timón R, Olcina G, González-Custodio A, Camacho-Cardenosa M, Camacho-Cardenosa A, Martínez Guardado I. Effects of 7-day intake of hydrogen-rich water on physical performance of trained and untrained subjects. *Biol Sport.* 2021 Jun;38(2):269-75. doi:10.5114/biolsport.2020.98625. Epub 2020 Oct 22. PMID: 34079172; PMCID: PMC8139351.

Chapter 9: Breathe 411

1. Garcia AJ, Ramirez JM. Keeping carbon dioxide in check. *Elife.* 2017 May 17;6:e27563. doi:10.7554/eLife.27563. PMID: 28513432; PMCID: PMC5435460.
2. Patel S, Miao JH, Yetiskul E, Anokhin A, Majmundar SH. Physiology, Carbon Dioxide Retention. 2022 Dec 26. *StatPearls.* Treasure Island (FL): StatPearls Publishing; 2024. PMID: 29494063.
3. Encyclopedia Britannica, "How Much Air Do You Breathe in a Lifetime?" https://www.britannica.com/video/253596/How-much-air-do-people-breathe-in-a-lifetime.
4. Ivanov KP. New data on the process of circulation and blood oxygenation in the lungs under physiological conditions. *Bull Exp Biol Med.* 2013 Feb;154(4):411-14. English, Russian. doi:10.1007/s10517-013-1963-1. PMID: 23486567.
5. Lefrançais E, Ortiz-Muñoz G, Caudrillier A, Mallavia B, Liu F, Sayah DM, Thornton EE, Headley MB, David T, Coughlin SR, Krummel MF, Leavitt AD, Passegué E, Looney MR. The lung is a site of platelet biogenesis and a reservoir for haematopoietic progenitors. *Nature.* 2017 Apr 6;544(7648):105-09. doi:10.1038/nature21706. Epub 2017 Mar 22. PMID: 28329764; PMCID: PMC5663284.
6. CDC. QuickStats: Percentage of Injury Deaths That Occurred in the Decedent's Home for the Five Most Common Causes of Injury Death—United States, 2016. *Weekly.* 2018 July 6;67(26):750. https://www.cdc.gov/mmwr/volumes/67/wr/mm6726a6.htm
7. Milroy CM. Deaths from Environmental Hypoxia and Raised Carbon Dioxide. *Acad Forensic Pathol.* 2018 Mar;8(1):2-7. doi:10.23907/2018.001. Epub 2018 Mar 7. PMID: 31240022; PMCID: PMC6474450.
8. Li D, Mabrouk OS, Liu T, Tian F, Xu G, Rengifo S, Choi SJ, Mathur A, Crooks CP, Kennedy RT, Wang MM, Ghanbari H, Borjigin J. Asphyxia-activated corticocardiac signaling accelerates onset of cardiac arrest. *Proc Natl Acad Sci.* 2015 Apr 21;112(16):E2073-82. doi:10.1073/pnas.1423936112.

Epub 2015 Apr 6. PMID: 25848007; PMCID: PMC4413312.

9. Giordano FJ. Oxygen, oxidative stress, hypoxia, and heart failure. *J Clin Invest.* 2005 Mar;115(3):500-08. doi:10.1172/JCI24408. PMID: 15765131; PMCID: PMC1052012.

Chapter 10: Breathe Assessment Tools

1. Szpilman D, Orlowski JP. Sports related to drowning. *Eur Respir Rev.* 2016 Sep;25(141):348-59. doi:10.1183/16000617.0038-2016. PMID: 27581833; PMCID: PMC9487220.

2. CO2 Tolerance Assessment. *Shift.* https://shiftadapt.com/breath -calculator.

Chapter 11: Troubleshooting Breathe

1. Jung JY, Kang CK. Investigation on the Effect of Oral Breathing on Cognitive Activity Using Functional Brain Imaging. *Healthcare* (Basel). 2021 May 29;9(6):645. doi:10.3390/healthcare9060645. PMID: 34072444; PMCID: PMC8228257.

2. Maydych V. The Interplay Between Stress, Inflammation, and Emotional Attention: Relevance for Depression. *Front Neurosci.* 2019 Apr 24;13:384. doi:10.3389/fnins.2019.00384. PMID: 31068783; PMCID: PMC6491771.

3. Russo MA, Santarelli DM, O'Rourke D. The physiological effects of slow breathing in the healthy human. *Breathe* (Sheff). 2017 Dec;13(4):298-309. doi:10.1183/20734735.009817. PMID: 29209423; PMCID: PMC5709795.

4. Roman MA, Rossiter HB, Casaburi R. Exercise, ageing and the lung. *European Respiratory Journal.* 2016 Nov;48(5)1471-86; doi:10.1183/13993003. 00347-2016.

5. Davies GA, Bolton CE. Age-related changes in the respiratory system. *Fillit HM,* Rockwood K, Young J, eds. *Brocklehurst's Textbook of Geriatric Medicine and Gerontology.* 8th ed. Philadelphia, PA: Elsevier; 2017:chap 17.

6. Vidotto LS, Carvalho CRF, Harvey A, Jones M. Dysfunctional breathing: what do we know? *J Bras Pneumol.* 2019 Feb 11;45(1):e20170347. doi:10.1590 /1806-3713/e20170347. PMID: 30758427; PMCID: PMC6534396.

7. Yackle K, Schwarz LA, Kam K, Sorokin JM, Huguenard JR, Feldman JL, Luo L, Krasnow MA. Breathing control center neurons that promote arousal in mice. *Science.* 2017 Mar 31;355(6332):1411-15. doi:10.1126/science. aai7984. Epub 2017 Mar 30. PMID: 28360327; PMCID: PMC5505554.

8. Moon SW, Leem AY, Kim YS, Lee JH, Kim TH, Oh YM, Shin H, Chang J, Jung JY; KOLD Study Group. Low serum lymphocyte level is associated with poor exercise capacity and quality of life in chronic obstructive pulmonary disease. *Sci Rep.* 2020 Jul 16;10(1):11700. doi:10.1038/s41598-020-68670-3. PMID: 32678181; PMCID: PMC7366616.

9. Bradley H, Esformes J. Breathing pattern disorders and functional movement. *Int J Sports Phys Ther.* 2014 Feb;9(1):28-39. PMID: 24567853; PMCID: PMC3924606.

10. Rodríguez-Molinero A, Narvaiza L, Ruiz J, Gálvez-Barrón C. Normal Respiratory Rate and Peripheral Blood Oxygen Saturation in the Elderly Population. *Journal of the American Geriatrics Society.* 2013;61:238-40. doi:10.1111/jgs.12580.

11. Shetty SR, Al Bayatti SW, Al-Rawi NH, Kamath V, Reddy S, Narasimhan S, Al Kawas S, Madi M, Achalli S, Bhat S. The effect of concha bullosa and nasal septal deviation on palatal dimensions: a cone beam computed tomography study. *BMC Oral Health.* 2021 Nov 23;21(1):607. doi:10.1186/s12903-021-01974-6. PMID: 34814910; PMCID: PMC8609805.

12. Yi-Fong Su V, Chou KT, Tseng CH, Kuo CY, Su KC, Perng DW, Chen YM, Chang SC. Mouth opening/breathing is common in sleep apnea and linked to more nocturnal water loss. *Biomed J.* 2023 Jun;46(3):100536. doi:10.1016/j.bj.2022.05.001. Epub 2022 May 10. PMID: 35552020; PMCID: PMC10209680.

13. Balasubramanian S, Vinayachandran D. Bioaerosols from mouth-breathing: Under-recognized transmissible mode in COVID-19? *Can Commun Dis Rep.* 2021 Jun 9;47(56):276-78. doi:10.14745/ccdr.v47i56a05. PMID: 34220352; PMCID: PMC8219058.

14. Stone, L. Are You Breathing? Do You Have Email Apnea? *Linda Stone Blog.* 2008 Feb. https://lindastone.net/2014/11/24/are-you-breathing-do-you-have-email-apnea.

Chapter 12: Breathe for the Win

1. Mooventhan A, Khode V. Effect of Bhramari pranayama and OM chanting on pulmonary function in healthy individuals: A prospective randomized control trial. *Int J Yoga.* 2014 Jul;7(2):104-10. doi:10.4103/0973-6131.133875. PMID: 25035619; PMCID: PMC4097894.

2. Voroshilov AP, Volinsky AA, Wang Z, Marchenko EV. Modified Qigong Breathing Exercise for Reducing the Sense of Hunger on an Empty Stomach. *J Evid Based Complementary Altern Med.* 2017 Oct;22(4):687-95. doi:10.1177/2156587217707143. Epub 2017 May 12. PMID: 28497701; PMCID: PMC5871281.

3. Yong MS, Lee YS, Lee HY. Effects of breathing exercises on resting metabolic rate and maximal oxygen uptake. *J Phys Ther Sci.* 2018 Sep;30(9):1173-75. doi:10.1589/jpts.30.1173. Epub 2018 Sep 4. PMID: 30214120; PMCID: PMC6127488.

4. Telles S, Sharma SK, Yadav A, Singh N, Balkrishna A. A comparative controlled trial comparing the effects of yoga and walking for overweight and

obese adults. *Med Sci Monit.* 2014 May 31;20:894-904. doi:10.12659/MSM.889805. PMID: 24878827; PMCID: PMC4051462.

5. Min J, Rouanet J, Martini AC, et al. Modulating heart rate oscillation affects plasma amyloid beta and tau levels in younger and older adults. *Sci Rep* 2023;13, 3967. doi:10.1038/s41598-023-30167-0.

6. Ahmad MA, Kareem O, Khushtar M, Akbar M, Haque MR, Iqubal A, Haider MF, Pottoo FH, Abdulla FS, Al-Haidar MB, Alhajri N. Neuroinflammation: A Potential Risk for Dementia. *Int J Mol Sci.* 2022 Jan 6;23(2):616. doi:10.3390/ijms23020616. PMID: 35054805; PMCID: PMC8775769.

7. Chen YF, Huang XY, Chien CH, Cheng JF. The Effectiveness of Diaphragmatic Breathing Relaxation Training for Reducing Anxiety. *Perspect Psychiatr Care.* 2017 Oct;53(4):329-36. doi:10.1111/ppc.12184. Epub 2016 Aug 23. PMID: 27553981.

8. Ma X, Yue ZQ, Gong ZQ, Zhang H, Duan NY, Shi YT, Wei GX, Li YF. The Effect of Diaphragmatic Breathing on Attention, Negative Affect and Stress in Healthy Adults. *Front Psychol.* 2017 Jun 6;8:874. doi:10.3389/fpsyg.2017.00874. PMID: 28626434; PMCID: PMC5455070.

9. Brown RP, Gerbarg PL. Sudarshan Kriya yogic breathing in the treatment of stress, anxiety, and depression: part I-neurophysiologic model. *J Altern Complement Med.* 2005 Feb;11(1):189-201. doi:10.1089/acm.2005.11.189. Erratum in: *J Altern Complement Med.* 2005 Apr;11(2):383-84. PMID: 15750381.

10. Ma X, Yue ZQ, Gong ZQ, Zhang H, Duan NY, Shi YT, Wei GX, Li YF. The Effect of Diaphragmatic Breathing on Attention, Negative Affect and Stress in Healthy Adults. *Front Psychol.* 2017 Jun 6;8:874. doi:10.3389/fpsyg.2017.00874. PMID: 28626434; PMCID: PMC5455070.

11. Sood R, Sood A, Wolf SL, Linquist BM, Liu H, Sloan JA, Satele DV, Loprinzi CL, Barton DL. Paced breathing compared with usual breathing for hot flashes. *Menopause.* 2013 Feb;20(2):179-84. doi:10.1097/gme.0b013e31826934b6. PMID: 22990758.

12. Zautra AJ, Fasman R, Davis MC, Craig ADB. The effects of slow breathing on affective responses to pain stimuli: an experimental study. *Pain.* 2010 Apr;149(1):12-18. doi:10.1016/j.pain.2009.10.001. Epub 2010 Jan 15. PMID: 20079569.

13. Mehling WE, Hamel KA, Acree M, Byl N, Hecht FM. Randomized, controlled trial of breath therapy for patients with chronic low-back pain. *Altern Ther Health Med.* 2005 Jul-Aug;11(4):44-52. PMID: 16053121.

14. American Migraine Foundation. Relaxation and Paced Breathing Exercises for Migraine. 2023 Sept 6. https://americanmigrainefoundation.org/resource-library/breathing-exercises-for-migraine.

15. Busch V, Magerl W, Kern U, Haas J, Hajak G, Eichhammer P. The effect of

deep and slow breathing on pain perception, autonomic activity, and mood processing—an experimental study. *Pain Med*. 2012 Feb;13(2):215-28. doi:10.1111/j.1526-4637.2011.01243.x. Epub 2011 Sep 21. PMID: 21939499.

16. Fang FC. Perspectives series: host/pathogen interactions. Mechanisms of nitric oxide-related antimicrobial activity. *J Clin Invest*. 1997 Jun 15;99(12):2818-25. doi:10.1172/JCI119473. PMID: 9185502; PMCID: PMC508130.

17. Mori H, Yamamoto H, Kuwashima M, Saito S, Ukai H, Hirao K, Yamauchi M, Umemura S. How does deep breathing affect office blood pressure and pulse rate? *Hypertens Res*. 2005 Jun;28(6):499-504. doi:10.1291/hypres .28.499. PMID: 16231755.

18. Jun HJ, Kim KJ, Nam KW, Kim CH. Effects of breathing exercises on lung capacity and muscle activities of elderly smokers. *J Phys Ther Sci*. 2016 Jun;28(6):1681-85. doi:10.1589/jpts.28.1681. Epub 2016 Jun 28. PMID: 27390394; PMCID: PMC4932035.

19. Carlson LE, Beattie TL, Giese-Davis J, Faris P, Tamagawa R, Fick LJ, Degelman ES, Speca M. Mindfulness-based cancer recovery and supportive-expressive therapy maintain telomere length relative to controls in distressed breast cancer survivors. *Cancer*. 2015;121:476-84. doi:10 .1002/cncr.29063.

20. Allen, Ruth M. "The health benefits of nose breathing." *Nursing in general practice*. 2015:40-42. http://hdl.handle.net/10147/559021.

21. Bahadoran Z, Carlström M, Mirmiran P, Ghasemi A. Nitric oxide: To be or not to be an endocrine hormone? *Acta Physiol* (Oxf). 2020 May;229(1):e13443. doi:10.1111/apha.13443. Epub 2020 Jan 26. PMID: 31944587.

22. Saura M, Zaragoza C, McMillan A, Quick RA, Hohenadl C, Lowenstein JM, Lowenstein CJ. An antiviral mechanism of nitric oxide: inhibition of a viral protease. *Immunity*. 1999 Jan;10(1):21-28. doi:10.1016/s1074-7613(00)80003-5. PMID: 10023767; PMCID: PMC7129050.

23. Akerström S, Mousavi-Jazi M, Klingström J, Leijon M, Lundkvist A, Mirazimi A. Nitric oxide inhibits the replication cycle of severe acute respiratory syndrome coronavirus. *J Virol*. 2005 Feb;79(3):1966-69. doi:10.1128/JVI.79.3.1966-1969.2005. PMID: 15650225; PMCID: PMC544093.

24. Lazar EE, Wills RB, Ho BT, Harris AM, Spohr LJ. Antifungal effect of gaseous nitric oxide on mycelium growth, sporulation and spore germination of the postharvest horticulture pathogens, Aspergillus niger, Monilinia fructicola and Penicillium italicum. *Lett Appl Microbiol*. 2008

Jun;46(6):688-92. doi:10.1111/j.1472-765X.2008.02373.x. Epub 2008 Apr 28. PMID: 18444976.

25. Schairer DO, Chouake JS, Nosanchuk JD, Friedman AJ. The potential of nitric oxide releasing therapies as antimicrobial agents. *Virulence.* 2012 May 1;3(3):271-79. doi:10.4161/viru.20328. Epub 2012 May 1. PMID: 22546899; PMCID: PMC3442839.

26. Lundberg JO, Settergren G, Gelinder S, Lundberg JM, Alving K, Weitzberg E. Inhalation of nasally derived nitric oxide modulates pulmonary function in humans. *Acta Physiol Scand.* 1996 Dec;158(4):343-47. doi:10.1046 /j.1365-201X.1996.557321000.x. PMID: 8971255.

27. Hord NG, Tang Y, Bryan NS. Food sources of nitrates and nitrites: the physiologic context for potential health benefits. *Am J Clin Nutr.* 2009 Jul;90(1):1-10. doi:10.3945/ajcn.2008.27131. Epub 2009 May 13. PMID: 19439460.

28. Kiani AK, Bonetti G, Medori MC, Caruso P, Manganotti P, Fioretti F, Nodari S, Connelly ST, Bertelli M. Dietary supplements for improving nitric-oxide synthesis. *J Prev Med Hyg.* 2022 Oct 17;63(2 Suppl 3):E239-E245. doi:10.15167/2421-4248/jpmh2022.63.2S3.2766. PMID: 36479475; PMCID: PMC9710401.

29. US Food and Drug Administration. Is Rinsing Your Sinuses with Neti Pots Safe? *Consumer Updates.* 2023 October 5. https://www.fda.gov/consumers /consumer-updates/rinsing-your-sinuses-neti-pots-safe.

30. Yamprasert R, Chanvimalueng W, Mukkasombut N, Itharat A. Ginger extract versus Loratadine in the treatment of allergic rhinitis: a randomized controlled trial. *BMC Complement Med Ther.* 2020 Apr 20;20(1):119. doi:10.1186/s12906-020-2875-z. PMID: 32312261; PMCID: PMC7171779.

31. Blanco-Salas J, Hortigón-Vinagre MP, Morales-Jadán D, Ruiz-Téllez T. Searching for Scientific Explanations for the Uses of Spanish Folk Medicine: A Review on the Case of Mullein (Verbascum, Scrophulariaceae). *Biology* (Basel). 2021 Jul 2;10(7):618. doi:10.3390/biology10070618. PMID: 34356473; PMCID: PMC8301161.

32. Turker A, Camper N. Biological activity of Common Mullein, a medicinal plant. *Journal of ethnopharmacology.* 2002;82:117-25. doi:10.1016/S0378-8741(02)00186-1.

33. Ghiya S. Alternate nostril breathing: a systematic review of clinical trials. *International Journal of Research in Medical Sciences.* 2017;5:3273. doi:10.18203 /2320-6012.ijrms20173523.

34. Balban MY, Neri E, Kogon MM, Weed L, Nouriani B, Jo B, Holl G, Zeitzer JM, Spiegel D, Huberman AD. Brief structured respiration practices enhance mood and reduce physiological arousal. *Cell Rep Med.* 2023 Jan

17;4(1):100895. doi:10.1016/j.xcrm.2022.100895. Epub 2023 Jan 10. PMID: 36630953; PMCID: PMC9873947.

35. Balban MY, Neri E, Kogon MM, Weed L, Nouriani B, Jo B, Holl G, Zeitzer JM, Spiegel D, Huberman AD. Brief structured respiration practices enhance mood and reduce physiological arousal. *Cell Rep Med.* 2023 Jan 17;4(1):100895. doi:10.1016/j.xcrm.2022.100895. Epub 2023 Jan 10. PMID: 36630953; PMCID: PMC9873947.

36. Breathing Exercises. *Wim Hof Method.* https://www.wimhofmethod.com /breathing-exercises.

37. Kopplin CS, Rosenthal L. The positive effects of combined breathing techniques and cold exposure on perceived stress: a randomised trial. *Curr Psychol.* 2022 Oct 7:1-13. doi:10.1007/s12144-022-03739-y. Epub ahead of print. PMID: 36248220; PMCID: PMC9540300.

38. Si S Çeli K A, Kılınç T. The effect of laughter yoga on perceived stress, burnout, and life satisfaction in nurses during the pandemic: A randomized controlled trial. *Complement Ther Clin Pract.* 2022 Nov;49:101637. doi:10.1016/j.ctcp.2022.101637. Epub 2022 Jul 5. PMID: 35810525; PMCID: PMC9254653.

39. Jerath R, Beveridge C, Barnes VA. Self-Regulation of Breathing as an Adjunctive Treatment of Insomnia. *Front Psychiatry.* 2019 Jan 29;9:780. doi:10.3389/fpsyt.2018.00780. PMID: 30761030; PMCID: PMC6361823.

40. Corrado J, Iftekhar N, Halpin S, Li M, Tarrant R, Grimaldi J, Simms A, O'Connor RJ, Casson A, Sivan M. HEART Rate Variability Biofeedback for Long COVID Dysautonomia (HEARTLOC): Results of a Feasibility Study. *Adv Rehabil Sci Pract.* 2024 Jan 28;13:27536351241227261. doi:10.1177 /27536351241227261. PMID: 38298551; PMCID: PMC10826406.

41. Lee YC, Lu CT, Cheng WN, Li HY. The Impact of Mouth-Taping in Mouth-Breathers with Mild Obstructive Sleep Apnea: A Preliminary Study. *Healthcare* (Basel). 2022 Sep 13;10(9):1755. doi:10.3390/healthcare10091755. PMID: 36141367; PMCID: PMC9498537.

42. LaComb C, Tandy R, Lee S, Young J, Navalta J. Oral versus Nasal Breathing during Moderate to High Intensity Submaximal Aerobic Exercise. *International Journal of Kinesiology and Sports Science.* 2017;5:8. doi:10.7575// aiac.ijkss.v.5n.1p.8.

43. Bahi C, Irrmischer M, Franken K, Fejer G, Schlenker A, Deijen J, Engelbregt H. Effects of conscious connected breathing on cortical brain activity, mood and state of consciousness in healthy adults. *Current Psychology.* 2023 Sep 8;43:10578-89. doi:10.1007/s12144-023-05119-6.

44. Londoño E. "Breathing Their Way to an Altered State." *New York Times,* Jan. 9, 2024.

Chapter 13: The Sleep-Drink-Breathe Nexus

1. Svensson S, Olin AC, Hellgren J. Increased net water loss by oral compared to nasal expiration in healthy subjects. *Rhinology.* 2006 Mar;44(1):74-77. PMID: 16550955.

index

Page numbers in *italics* indicate illustrations.

acetaminophen, 66
acid reflux, 84, 112
acute viral hepatitis, 111
adenosine in, 22, 51, 84, 90
adrenaline, 84, 85, 222, 229, 250
Advil PM, 66
aerobic exercise, 178–79, 202, 227
age
    biological vs. chronological, 141
    declining lung function and, 9
    heart rate variability and, 228
    respiratory rates and, 198
    respiratory system and, 193–94
    water needs and, 146, 161
Agni Pran, 224
air hunger, 169, 170, 174, 176
air quality, 88–89
airflow strength, 182–83, 185
Airofit Pro, 182, 216, 245
airways
    blockage of, 69, 174, 199
    hydration and, 238
    mucus in, 170, 176, 219
alcohol, 85, 93
    breathing and, 228
    sleep and, 36, 40, 65, 73
    Sleep-Drink-Breathe Plan and, 243,
        253, 259, 267, 269
    urinary frequency and, 117–18
    vasopressin and, 85, 118, 160
alertness breathing, 222–24, 229, 251
alkaline water, 159
allergies, 178, 199, 213–14
alternate-nostril breathing, 221,
    259, 266

alveoli, 170–71, *172*, 193, 238
Alzheimer's Disease, 127, 207
Ambien, 66
American Academy of Sleep Medicine,
    226
American Migraine Foundation, 210
amino acids, 26, 229, 230
amitriptyline, 112
ANS (autonomic nervous system), 4–5,
    208, 229
anti-inflammatories, 66, 76, 143, 159, 220,
    229–30
antibodies, 76
antidepressants, 40, 112
antidiuretic hormone. *See* vasopressin
antihistamines, 66–67, 215
antioxidants, 135, 143, 155, 213, 229, 230
anxiety, 191
    breathing and, 192, 194, 208, 221,
        223
    sleep and, 18, 51, 53, 63, 72, 81, 92
Apollo Neuro, 47
appetite, 78, 233
appetite-control breathing, 225
arthritis, 8, 112, 143, 190, 208
asparagus, 112, 155
asphyxiation, 173–75
asthma, 174, 182, 194, 197, 213
atherosclerosis, 127
autonomic nervous system (ANS), 4–5,
    208, 229
Avatar, 175
avocados, 133, *134,* 155
awakeness, accepting, 92–93, 94,
    260, 267

back pain, 196, 203, 210, 269
bears (chronotype), 55–56, 57
  cortisol of, 57, 238
  dinner time of, 84
  ideal bedtime of, 59, 82, 253, 259
  ideal wake time of, 59, 81, 243, 249,
    255, 262
  inner alarms of, 58
  napping and, 91, 265
  Sleep-Drink-Breathe Plan and, 243
    Week 1, 249, 250, 251, 252, 253
    Week 2, 255, 256, 257, 258, 259
    Week 3, 262, 263, 264, 265, 266, 267
bedrooms, 87–89, 94, 244
beer, 117–18. *See also* alcohol
belly breathing, 217, 233, 239
benign prostatic hyperplasia (BPH), 116,
  119, 120, 121
beta blockers, 66
biological age vs. chronological age, 141
bladder, 116, 119, 120, 129
bloating, 133–35, 138, 154, 160
blood, 99, 168, 172, 229
blood oxygen test, 181
blood pressure
  alternate-nostril breathing and, 221
  anxiety and, 63
  cortisol and, 211
  dehydration and, 107, 126, 138
  garlic and, 229
  high, 50, 66, 151, 190, 191
  low, 126, 138
  magnesium and, 156
  overhydration and, 102
  sleep and, 4, 22, 25
  vigorous exercise and, 85
blood sodium, normal range for, 131
blood volume, 99, 102, 104, 106, 239
body mass index (BMI), 52, 56, 142, 206, 207
body temperature, 4, 22, 85, 100, 106, 237
body weight
  breathing and, 206–7
  heart rate variability and, 228
  hydration and, 127, 142, 146, 147, 161–62
  sleep and, 52, 77–78, 81

box (4-4-4-4) breathing, 221, 238, 250,
  252, 264, 268
BPH (benign prostatic hyperplasia), 116,
  119, 120, 121
brain, 99, 144
  adenosine in, 22, 51, 84, 90
  aerobic exercise and, 179
  breathing and, 5, 195
  cerebrospinal fluid and, 100
  dehydration and, 101, 102, 104
  dreams and, 28
  microsleep and, 173
  neuroplasticity of, 21
  osmoregulation and, 100–101, *101*
  overhydration and, 102, 126, 138
  oxygen deprivation and, 174–75
  quenching and, 104
  release of vasopressin, 85
  sleep and, 25, 26, 31–32, 33, 78–79, 236
  sodium levels and, 131
  waking up and, 84
brain fog, 31, 81, 103, 116, 199
Brain Plasticity Theory, 21
breastfeeding, 147
breath of fire, 224
breathing, 2–3, 4–5, 8–9
  4-7-8 breathing technique, 64, 221,
    238, 254, 268
  age and, 193–94, 198
  alertness, 222–24, 229, 251
  alternate-nostril, 221, 259, 266
  appetite-control, 225
  assessment of, 178–84, 185
  belly, 217, 233, 239
  benefits of good breathing, 206–11
  box (4-4-4-4), 221, 238, 250, 252, 264,
    268
  breathwork and, 185, 201, 230–32,
    232n, 234
  calming, 220–22
  cognitive performance and, 189
  compromised immunity and, 191–92
  congestion and, 213–15, 214n
  diaphragm and, 5, 169, 171, 191–92,
    193, 215–17, 233

diaphragmatic, 208, 225, 231, 238
exercise and, 228–29
fast, 197–98
heart rate variability and, 228–29
heart-supporting foods and
    supplements for, 229–30
holding breaths, 201–2, 203
holotropic, 231–32
horizontal, 196
importance of, 166–68, *167*, 192–94
interconnectedness between
    hydration, sleep, and, 235–36,
    237–39
modified Qigong, 225, 252, 258, 265
mouth, 198–201, 203, 214, 228, 239, 261
mouth tape and, 226–27
nasal, 212–13, 226, 227, 228, 233, 251, 264
oral, 189, 228
phlegm and, 219–20
posture and, 218–19, 233, 239, 245, 258
process of, 169–72, 176
Qigong, 206
during REM, 25
resonant, 225–26, 261, 268
shallow, 194–96
in Sleep-Drink-Breathe Plan, 245,
    247–48, 269
    Week 1, 250, 251–53, 254
    Week 2, 256–58, 259, 261
    Week 3, 263, 264, 265, 266, 268
sleep-inducing, 225–26
sleep issues and, 191
stress, inflammation, and, 189–90
survival time without, 173–75
thoracic, 194
vertical, 196
yogic, 206
breathwork, 185, 201, 230–32, 232n, 234
Breus, Michael, 8, 30
    Extreme Performance Training and,
        169–70
    The Power of When, 36, 55n
    The Sleep Doctor's Diet Plan, 52
    Wim Hoff controlled hyperventilation
        method and, 223, *223*

Brigham Young study, 52
bright light therapy, 71
bronchi, 170, 172, 173, 238
bronchioles, 170, 171, 172, 219, 238
brussels sprouts, 133, 155

caffeine
    dehydration and, 118
    diuretic effect of, 134
    intake, timing of, 83–84
    before napping, 90–91
    sleep and, 40, 73
    Sleep-Drink-Breathe Plan and, 243
        Week 1, 250, 253
        Week 2, 256, 259
        Week 3, 263, 267
    sleep stages and, 65
    urinary frequency and, 118
calcium, 100, 135, 140, 156
California Institute of Technology, 104
calming breathing techniques, 220–22
cancer, 80, 136, 141
cannabis, 40, 66
capsaicin, 230
carbon dioxide, 5, 69, 169, 190
    breathwork and, 230
    circulation and, 227
    exhalation and, 166, *167*, 167–68, 171,
        176
    hydration and, 239
    overdose death, 174
carbon dioxide tolerance test, 183–84
carbonated water, 160
cardiorespiratory coupling, 190
cardiovascular disease, 30, 50, 62
cardiovascular system, 99, 190, 191
Carnegie Mellon University study, 50
carrots, 11, 155
cats, 112, 214
cayenne pepper, 230
CBD products, 66
celery, 135, 155, 213
Centers for Disease Control, 136, 145, 174
central sleep apnea, 69
cerebrospinal fluid, 26, 100

children
  amount of sleep needed by, 36
  mouth breathing and, 199
  respiratory rate of, 198
chronic fatigue syndrome, 69–70
chronic inflammation, 190
  breathing and, 203, 208
  hydration and, 8, 143
  sleep and, 77
chronic obstructive pulmonary disease
    (COPD), 3, 174, 178, 181, 197, 208
chronological age vs. biological age, 141
chronoquiz.com, 72
chronorhythm. *See* circadian rhythm
chronotypes, 36, 55
  dinner time and, 84–85
  napping and, 91
  Sleep-Drink-Breathe Plan and, 243
    Week 1, 249, 250, 251, 252, 253
    Week 2, 255, 256, 257, 258, 259
    Week 3, 262, 263, 264, 266, 267
  types of, 55–60, 72–73, 81–82, 93, 243.
    See also specific chronotypes
cigarette smoking, 66
cimetidine, 112
circadian rhythm, 22, 80, 189
  chronotypes and, 55–58, 82, 243
  hypothalamus and, 100
  interference of light from devices
    with, 40, 253
  kidneys and, 85, 115, 132
  living out of sync with, 55–59
  napping and, 94
  oversleeping and, 61–62
  Sleep-Drink-Breathe Plan and, 243
  sleeping in and, 60–61
  wake time and, 81
circadian rhythm sleep-wake disorders,
    69, 71
circulation, 160–61, 162, 191, 227, 228,
    233, 266
circulatory system, 8, 106–7, 227, 228
cirrhosis, 111
classical conditioning, 149
clitoris, 144, 211

coconut water, 135
Coenzyme Q10 (CoQ10), 229
coffee, 121
  before napping, 90–91, 265
  Sleep-Drink-Breathe Plan and, 250,
    256, 263, 264, 265
  urinary frequency and, 118
  See also caffeine
cognitive behavioral therapy, 71
cognitive function, 126, 143–44, 189,
    209, 221
cold (illness), 147, 213
colon, 99, 126, 140
compliance, 11
congestion, 88, 198, 199, 213–15, 214n, 237
consistency in sleep-wake patterns, 60,
    81–83
constipation, 100, 112, 126, 138
continuous positive airway pressure
    (CPAP) machine, 71, 157,
    200–201, 226
Cooper, Bradley, 131
COPD (chronic obstructive pulmonary
    disease), 3, 174, 178, 181, 197, 208
CoQ10 (Coenzyme Q10), 229
cortisol, 189, 211
  breathing and, 203, 208, 222
  chronotypes and, 57, 59, 82, 238
  hydration and, 237
  inflammation and, 190
  panic attacks and, 194
  postprandial dip in, 90
  serotonin and, 86
  sleep and, 4, 22, 23, 33, 63, 191
  Sleep-Drink-Breathe Plan and, 250
  vigorous exercise and, 85
  wake time and, 81, 84
coughing, controlled, 219–20, 256, 263
countertop water filters, 158
COVID-19 pandemic, 18, 92, 181, 193,
    199, 226
CPAP (continuous positive airway
    pressure) machine, 71, 157,
    200–201, 226
cramps, leg, 70, 125, 237

creativity, 79
cyclic hyperventilating, 222–23, 251, 253,
    257, 259, 264, 265, 266
cyclic sighing, 221–22, 256–57, 264

Darwin, Charles, 21
DBPs (disinfectant byproducts), 136–37
deep vein thrombosis, 134
dehydration, 8, 102–3, 108, 239
    bad habits responsible for, 128–30,
        132–35, *133*, 138, 149
    brain and, 101, 102, 104
    caffeine and, 118
    circulation and, 160
    consequences of, 106–7, 124–27, 138
    constipation and, 100, 126, 138
    definition of, 102, 125, 138
    gulping signal and, 104, 105, 106
    heart rate variability and, 229
    leg cramps and, 237
    mouth breathing and, 203
    pinch test for, 112–13, 120–21
    thirst cue and, 104–5
    Thirst Discomfort Scale for, 113–14
Dement, William, 31
dementia, 67, 141, 143, 200, 208
depression, 53, 62, 68, 72, 103
deviated septum, 199, 214n
diabetes, 68, 213
    chronic inflammation and, 8, 143
    hydration and, 127, 141, 147, 151
    sleep and, 30, 50, 62
    stress and, 208
    urinary frequency and, 116, 120, 121
diaphragm, 5, 169, 171, 191–92, 193,
    215–17, 233
diaphragmatic breathing, 208, 225, 231,
    238
diarrhea, 103, 147, 151, 152
diary. *See* hydration diary; sleep diary
diet, 51, 147, 155, 225
digestion, 154, 265
digestive process, 140
digestive system, 99–100
dinner time, 84–85, 252, 258, 266

diphenhydramine antihistamines, 66–67
disco naps, 89
disinfectant byproducts (DBPs), 136–37
distilled water, 157, 162, 214
diuretics, 103, 134–35
dizziness, 107, 126, 151, 169, 197
Dmitrieva, Natalia, 141
dogs, 112
dolphins (chronotype), 57, *57*, 58–60, 71,
    237
    accepting awakeness, 92, 93
    body mass index of, 57
    cortisol of, 57, 82, 238
    dinner time of, 84
    ideal bedtime of, 59–60, 82, 253, 259
    ideal wake time of, 59–60, 82, 243,
        249, 255, 262
    napping and, 91
    resonant breathing and, 225–26
    Sleep-Drink-Breathe Plan and, 243
        Week 1, 249, 250, 251, 252, 253
        Week 2, 255, 256, 257, 258, 259
        Week 3, 262, 263, 264, 266, 267
dopamine, 4, 104, 224
dreams, 26, 27–29, 53
drinking. *See* hydration
drinking containers, 137
drowsiness, 22, 32, 45, 51

electrolytes
    dehydration and, 101, 103, 107, 124, 126
    extreme sickness and, 152
    osmoregulation and, 100, 108, 111
    water infused with, 124, 132, 147,
        150–51
electronic mouthpieces, 216
electronic reminder devices, 219, 245
endocrine system, 102, 132
endurance/elevation training masks,
    216, 245
energy
    breathing and, 167, *167*, 171, 208–9,
        222, 233
    dehydration and, 125, 138
    sleep and, 51–52, 77–78

Energy Conservation Theory, 19–20
Environmental Protection Agency, 88
Environmental Working Group (EWG),
    135–36
erectile dysfunction, 80, 144
essential naps, 89
European Respiration Journal, 193
exercise
    aerobic, 178–79, 202, 227
    bears (chronotype) and, 56
    breathing and, 228–29
    dolphins (chronotype) and, 57
    electrolyte powder and, 151–52
    hydration and, 146, 147
    lions (chronotype) and, 56
    sleep and, 51, 77
    Sleep-Drink-Breathe Plan and, 243,
        269
        Week 1, 253
        Week 2, 255, 258, 259
        Week 3, 266, 267
    timing of, 85–86, 93
    wolves (chronotype) and, 82
exhalation, 166–67
    breathwork and, 230
    carbon dioxide and, 166, *167,* 167–68,
        171, 176
    posture and, 233
    sleep and, 238
    Sleep-Drink-Breathe Plan and
        Week 1, 250, 251, 252, 254
        Week 2, 256, 257–58, 259, 261
        Week 3, 263
    testing, 182
expiration. *See* exhalation
Extreme Performance Training (XPT),
    169–70

falling sensation during sleep, 24–25
fatigue, 10, 19, 67, 69, 89, 91, 125
faucet-mounted water filters, 158
filters, water, 157–59
fish, 229
flu, 147, 213
Fogg, BJ, 150

food
    chronotypes and, 56
    drinking with, 154
    heart-supporting, 229–30
    sleep deprivation and, 29
    in Sleep-Drink-Breathe Plan, 243
        Week 1, 252, 253
        Week 2, 258, 259
        Week 3, 266, 267
    spicy, 65, 84
    water content of, 155, 162
Food and Drug Administration, 151,
    156, 214
Frontiers in Neurology, 51
fulfillment naps, 89

GABA (gamma-aminobutyric acid), 23
GALT (gut-associated mucosal tissue), 140
Gardner, Randy, 31
garlic, 229
gas exchange, 171, 176, 218
    aerobic exercise and, 202
    diaphragm in, 216
    heat and, 267
    hydration and, 228
    obstructive sleep apnea and, 200
    phlegm and, 219
gate pose, 217, *217,* 263
Gatorade, 151, 152
Gensler, Zach, 33
George III, 112
Georgia Highway Patrol, 32
ghrelin, 22, 33, 52, 78
ginger, 215
ginkgo biloba, 230
Glamour, 130, 131
glucose, 22, 99, 172
    breathing and, 167, *167,* 171, 176
    during REM, 26
glycogen, 51
glymphatic system, 26, 64, 100, 236
Godfather, The, 173
Grof, Stanislav, 231–32
growth hormone, 20, 25, 64, 213
gulping signal, 104, 105, 106

gums, 112–13
gut
    breathing and, 4, 172
    hydration and, 104, 105, 107, 140, 154
gut-associated mucosal tissue (GALT), 140

habits, 128, 257
haloacetic acids, 136
Hamilton, Laird, 169, 170
harnesses, strap-on, 218, 245
headaches, 4, 27, 103, 126, 138, 144, 210
healthspan, 141
heart, 80, 99, 174, 190, 228, 229–30
heart attack, 174, 197–98, 229
heart disease
    chronic inflammation and, 143, 190
    hydration and, 127, 141, 147
    sleep and, 68, 200
    stress and, 208
    water retention and, 134
heart failure, 141
heart rate, 160
    anxiety and, 63
    breathing and, 190, 191, 221, 222–23
    cortisol and, 211
    exercise and, 85, 178–79
    healthy resting, 63
    hypothalamus and, 100
    panic attacks and, 194
    sleep and, 4, 25
    wolves (chronotype) and, 81
heart rate variability (HRV), 46, 201,
        228–29
heat, 267
hemoglobin, 168, 171, 181, 227
Hoff, Wim, 8, 223, *223*
holding breath test, 180, 184
holotropic breathing, 231–32
homeostasis, 5, 6, 9, 14, 110
    breathing and, 167–68, 203
    osmoregulation and, 100–102, *101*
horizontal breathing, 196
hot flashes, 209
HRV (heart rate variability), 46, 201,
        228–29

Hu, David, 119
humidity, 88–89, 244
hunger
    breathing and, 206
    hydration and, 142
    hypothalamus and, 100
    overactive thyroid and, 116
    sleep deprivation and, 33
    Sleep-Drink-Breathe Plan and, 251–52,
        258, 265
hydration, 8, 73, 100–103, 108, 125, 168
    assessment of, 110–14, 120–21
    benefits of, 140–45
    body's systems for, 4
    circulation and, 160–61, 162, 228
    cognition and, 126, 143–44
    congestion and, 215
    estimating water needs for, 145–48,
        161–62
    exercise and, 146
    food and, 154, 162
    forgetting, 128, 149
    habit, establishing a, 148–50
    importance of, 99–100
    interconnectedness between sleep,
        breathing, and, 235–36, 237, 238–39
    lifespan and, 141
    before meals, 142
    mistaking bloat for, 133–35
    multipliers, 150–52
    osmoregulation and, 100–102, *101*
    sex and, 44
    sipping and, 153, 162
    in Sleep-Drink-Breathe Plan, 243,
        245, 247
        Week 1, 249, 250, 251, 252, 253, 254
        Week 2, 255, 256, 257, 258–59, 260
        Week 3, 262, 264, 265, 266, 267, 268
    social media "challenges" relating to, 131
    survival time without, 105–7, 108, 173
    urine and, 101, *101*, 102, 106, 110, 111,
        117, 132–33
    water choice for, 156–57, 162
    See also dehydration; overhydration;
        underhydration

hydration diary in Sleep-Drink-Breathe
    Plan, 247
  Week 1, 249, 250, 251, 252
  Week 2, 255, 256, 257, 258, 260
  Week 3, 262, 264, 265, 266, 268
hydrogen water, 159–60
hypernatremia, 151
hypersomnia, 62
hypersomnolence, 69–70
hyperventilation, controlled, 175,
    222–24, 232
  cyclic, 222–23, 251, 253, 257, 259, 264,
    265, 266
  respiratory rate and, 197
  skull-shining breath, 224, 257–58, 259,
    264, 265, 266
  Wim Hoff method, 223, *223*
hypnic jerks, 24
hyponatremia, 131–32
hypothalamus, 4, 71, 100–101, *101*, 102
hypothalamus-pituitary complex, 102
hypoventilation, 69

ICSD- 3 (*International Classification of
    Sleep Disorders*), 68
immune system and immunity
  breathing and, 191–92, 203, 233
  hydration and, 143
  sleep and, 25, 33, 50, 76, 77, 93
incontinence, 129
indomethacin, 112
Indonesia hydration color chart, 111
infants, amount of sleep needed
    by, 36
inflammation
  anti-inflammatories and, 66, 76, 143,
    159, 220, 229–30
  breathing and, 207–8, 233
  chronic. *See* chronic inflammation
  hydration and, 100, 127, 138, 143, 159
  sleep and, 33, 51, 72, 76–77
  stress and, 189–90
inhalation, 166–67, 169, 176
  breathwork and, 230
  oxygen and, 166, 167, *167*, 170–71, 176

posture and, 233
sleep and, 238
Sleep-Drink-Breathe Plan and
  Week 1, 250, 251, 254
  Week 2, 256, 257, 259, 261
  Week 3, 263
  testing, 182
insomnia, 63, 68, 245
  anxiety-related, 226–27
  breathing and, 191, 225
  cognitive behavioral therapy
    for, 71
  COVID-19 pandemic and, 92
  depression and, 62
  napping and, 89
  nicotine and, 66
  overactive thyroid and, 116
  rates, increase in, 18
  stress and, 237
inspiration. *See* inhalation
intercostal muscles, 5, 173, 182, 194, 216,
    263
*International Classification of Sleep
    Disorders* (ICSD- 3), 68
iron, 71, 156
irritable bowel syndrome, 112
ischemic strokes, 29

jaw clenching, 70, 71
jet lag, 69, 71, 129
joint pain, 127
journaling, 87, 253
jumping, 227–28

kapalbhati, 224, 231
kidney disease
  hydration and, 103, 127, 131, 134, 138,
    147, 151
  sleep and, 68
kidney stones, 112, 116, 126, 147
kidneys, 160
  alcoholic beverages and, 118
  balancing of pH, 159
  circadian rhythm of, 85, 115, 132
  diabetes and, 116

hydration and, 102, 107, 131
osmoregulation and, 100, 101, *101*
sleep and, 236
urine color and, 110–11

L-arginine, 135, 213, 229
laughter yoga, 224, 264
learning, sleep and, 78–79
leg cramps, 70, 125, 237
leptin, 52, 78, 207
Life Gives to the Giver (Polish), 7
lifespan, 54, 79–80, 141, 210
light from devices, 40, 86, 89, 253, 260
lions (chronotype), 56, *57*
  accepting awakeness, 92, 93
  body mass index of, 56
  cortisol of, 57, 238
  dinner time of, 84
  ideal bedtime of, 59, 82, 253, 259
  ideal wake time of, 59, 81, 243, 249,
    255, 262
  inner alarms of, 58
  napping and, 91, 265
  Sleep-Drink-Breathe Plan and, 243
    Week 1, 249, 250, 251, 252, 253
    Week 2, 255, 256, 257, 258, 259
    Week 3, 262, 263, 264, 265, 266, 267
Liquid I.V. (hydration multiplier), 152
liver, 4, 107, 136, 160, 167, 172
liver disease, 111, 134
LMNT (hydration multiplier), 152
locus coeruleus, 195
lung disease, 141
lungs, 5, 29, 172–73, 176, 218
  age and, 9, 193
  alcohol and, 228
  assessing, 179, 182–83
  in breathing, 169, 170, 171
  heart-supporting foods and
    supplements and, 229–30
  lobes of, 195–96
  phlegm and, 219
  strength of, 9, 179
lymph nodes, 76, 191–92, 196
lymphatic system, 26, 100, 107, 191–92

Mackenzie, Brian, 183
magnesium, 71, 100, 111, 133, 156, 230, 245
magnesium deficiency, 134, 135
makeup, removing, 87
mangos, 111, 155
masks, endurance/elevation training,
  216, 245
meals, 65, 252, 258, 266
medications, 66, 111–12, 147
meditation, 230, 260
Mediterranean diet, 155
medulla oblongata, 5, 169
melatonin, 4, 22, 245
melons, 133, 135, 155
memory consolidation process, 26, 28
mental performance, 126, 209
metabolic rate, 206–7
microbiome, 140, 172
microsleep, 173
migraines, 126
Mihavecz, Andreas, 105–6, 173
mineral water, 140, 156, 162, 265
MIT, 79
modified Qigong breathing, 225, 252,
  258, 265
mood, 100, 103
mouth breathing, 198–201, 203, 214, 228,
  239, 261
mouth guards, 71
mouth tape, 226–27, 245, 261, 268
mucosal tissue, 140, 193
mucus
  in airways, 170, 176
  clearing, 219–20, 245, 256
  COVID and, 193
  excess, 196
  gut, 99, 140
  hydration and, 238
  in mouths, 170, 176
  nasal, 170, 176, 212, 214–15, 233, 237
mullein, 220, 245
multipliers, hydration, 150–52
muscle cramps, 103, 197
muscle mass, 77–78
Muse S Headband, 47

N-Acetyl cysteine (NAC), 230
nadi shodhana pranayama, 221
nanoplastics, 137, 138
napping, 65, 89–91, 94, 265
narcolepsy, 62, 69
nasal breathing, 212–13, 226, 227, 228, 233, 251, 264
nasal dilators, 215
nasal irrigation, 214
National Academy of Medicine, 145
National Highway Traffic Safety Administration, 32
National Institutes of Health, 52, 141
National Sleep Foundation, 8, 36
natural killer cells, 50
net-zero liquids, 118, 121, 160
neti pot, 214
neurological performance deficit, 32–33
New York Times, 231
newborns, 36, 198
nicotine, 62, 66, 73, 243, 253, 259, 267
Nightmare on Elm Street, A, 28–29
nitrate, 213
nitric oxide (NO), 212–13, 226, 229, 233
nocturnal leg cramps, 70, 237
NSAIDs (nonsteroidal anti-inflammatory drugs), 66
nutrient absorption, 154
nuts, 155

obesity, 29, 50, 52, 62, 68
obstructive sleep apnea (OSA), 29, 52, 62, 69, 200, 226
Ohio State University study, 32
older adults, 90, 103, 117, 129–30, 150, 198
omega-3 fatty acids, 229
oral appliances, 71
oral breathing, 189, 228
orgasms, 210–11, 233
OSA (obstructive sleep apnea). *See* obstructive sleep apnea (OSA)
osmoregulation, 100–102, *101*
Oura Ring, 46, 245
overactive thyroid, 116

overhydration, 102, 126, 130–32, 138
oversleeping, 61–62
oxidative stress, 33, 143, 189, 206–7, 208, 230
oxygen, 5, 69, 169, 190, 194, 208, 226
breathwork and, 230
circulation and, 160, 227
cognition and, 209
deprivation, 173–75
exercise and, 179, 227, 228
hydration and, 99, 106, 200, 239
inhalation and, 166, 167, *167,* 170–71, 176
Sleep-Drink-Breathe Plan and, 264

pain, 66–67, 116, 127, 196, 198, 210, 269
panic attacks, 178, 184, 194, 195, 197
parasomnia, 70
parasympathetic nervous system, 9, 47, 189, 208, 227
parsley, 135
peaches, 134, 155
peak flow devices, 182, 245
peppers, 155, 230
Petrović, Branko, 175
phenazopyridine, 111
phlegm. *See* mucus
physical performance, 126, 138, 160
physiological sighing, 221–22
pinch test, 112–13, 120–21
pineal gland, 4, 22
pitchers, water filter, 158–59
pituitary gland, 101, *101,* 102
plastic bottles/containers, 137, 138
pneumonia, 178, 181, 194, 197
Polish, Joe, 7
polysomnography. *See* sleep study
polyuria, 116
posture, 218–19, 233, 239, 245, 258, 259
potassium, 133, 156
potassium deficiency, 134, 135
Power-Down Hour, 86–87, 243, 253, 260–61, 267–68

Power of When, The (Breus), 36, 55n
pregnancy, 116, 133, 147
preschoolers, amount of sleep needed
    by, 36
Primal Hydration (hydration multiplier),
    152
proactive naps, 89
propofol, 112
prostate, enlarged, 116, 119, 120, 121
protein, 99, 154
pulmonary embolism, 178, 197
pulse, 25, 46, 181
pulse oximeters, 181
pure water, 157

Qigong breathing, 206
quality of life, 6, 140, 141
quenching, 104–5

rats, 30, 173, 174
recovery naps, 89
Reece, Gabby, 169–70
rehydration, 104–5
REM, 25–27, 34, 64–65, 84, 236
    cannabis and, 66
    creativity and, 79
    lifespan and, 54
    light from devices in interfering
        with, 40
    medications and, 66
    respiratory rate during, 238
    stress and, 53
    vigorous exercise and, 85
REM rebound, 27, 66
resonant breathing, 225–26, 261, 268
respiration. *See* breathing
respiration drive, 168, 169, 175
respiratory rate, 25, 182, 197–98,
    237–38
respiratory rate test, 178, 184
respiratory system, 190, 193–94
restless legs syndrome, 70
Restorative Theory, 20–21
riboflavin. *See* vitamin B12
ribs, 5, 171, 193, 216

rifampin, 111
Ross, John J., 31

salmon, 155, 229
satiety signal, 104
sauna, 267
school-age children, amount of sleep
    needed by, 36
Science, 194–95
SCN (suprachiasmatic nucleus), 4
screen apnea, 201, 264, 265
sedative-hypnotic drugs, 66
sedentary lifestyle, 134, 146, 160,
    202, 219
self- reported quality assessment of
    sleep, 41–45
self-reported thirst discomfort rating,
    113–14
senna, 112
serotonin, 23, 86, 172, 264
sexual activity, 80
    breathing and, 210–11, 233
    hydration and, 144
    sleep and, 80
Shields, Brooke, 130–31
shift-work sleep disorder, 69
short sleep, 50, 51, 54, 65, 132, 133
shortness of breath test, 178–79, 185
sighing, cyclic, 221–22, 256–57, 264
simhasana, 231
sipping, 153, 162
sitting, breathing and, 218–19, 233
Skene's glands, 144
skin, dehydration and, 107, 112–13,
    120–21, 127
skin turgor test
    for dehydration, 113
    Sleep-Drink-Breathe Plan and, 269
        pre-plan self-testing, 247
        Week 1, 249, 250, 251, 252
        Week 2, 255, 256, 258
        Week 3, 262, 264, 266
skincare routine at night, 87
skull-shining breath, 224, 257–58, 259,
    264, 265, 266

sleep, 2–3, 4, 23–24
  anxiety and, 18, 51, 53, 63, 72, 81, 92
  assessment, 25, 27, 36, 37–48, *38*, 48
  bedtime and, 82, 83
  benefits of good sleep, 76–80, 93
  better, tips for, 6–8
    accepting awakeness, 92–93, 94,
      260, 267
    consistency, 60, 81–83
    environment, 40, 87–89, 94
    napping, 89–91, 94
    shifting activities, 83–87, 93–94
  breathing and, 225–26, 239
  circadian rhythm and, 55–59
  COVID-19 pandemic and, 18
  death and, 29
  dehydration and, 132–33, *133*
  disorders, 18, 23, 67–71, 73, 80, 191. *See*
    also specific sleep disorders
  dreams during. *See* dreams
  freaking out about, 63–64
  habits disrupting, 64–67, 73
  interconnectedness between
    hydration, breathing, and, 7,
    235–36, 237–38
  oversleeping, 61–62
  playing catch-up, 60–62
  poor
    consequences of, 50–54, 72, 237
    hoping it goes away on its own, 67–71
  processes creating, 21–23, 34
  quality of, 34, 40–45, 48, 62
  quantity, 36–37, 40, 48, 50
  sensation of falling during, 24–25
  sex and, 80
  in Sleep-Drink-Breathe Plan, 243,
    244–45, 246–47, 269
    Week 1, 249, 250, 251, 252, 253–54
    Week 2, 255, 256, 257, 258, 260
    Week 3, 262, 263, 264–65
  stages of, 24–27, 34, 64–65, 77, 79, 236,
    237. *See also* REM
  theories about, 19–21
  urine and, 132
  vigorous exercise and, 85

Sleep (journal), 92
sleep apnea, 8, 69, 191, 238
  at-home test for, 71
  death and, 29, 200–201
  mouth breathing and, 199
  obstructive. *See* obstructive sleep
    apnea (OSA)
sleep cycles, 24–27, 34, 37, 65
sleep deprivation, 29–33, 173
  brain function and, 31–32
  chronic, 30, 34, 60, 89
  death and, 29–30
  heart rate variability and, 229
  neurological performance deficit
    with, 32–33
  parenthood and, 30
  physical pain and, 66–67
  PTSD sufferers and, 28
  risk factors of, 32–33
  severe, 31–33
  thirst and, 236
sleep diary, 37–40, *38*, 48, 70
  self-reported, 39–40
  Sleep-Drink-Breathe Plan and, 245,
    246–47, 249, 255, 260, 267
Sleep Doctor's Diet Plan, The (Breus), 52
Sleep-Drink-Breathe Plan, 11–12, 148,
  241–69
  changes after, 268–69
  daily times in, 242–43
  mid-morning, 242, 243, 250, 256–57,
    263–64
  post-lunch, 242, 243, 251–52, 257–58,
    264–65
  Power-Down Hour in, 86–87, 243, 253,
    260–61, 267–68
  pre-bedtime, 243, 253–54, 259–61,
    267–68
  pre-dinner, 243, 252–53, 258–59, 266–67
  preparing for, 244–48
  upon waking, 236, 242, 243, 249–50,
    255–56
  Week 1, 249–54
  Week 2, 255–61
  Week 3, 262–68

sleep drive, 21–22, 23, 34, 168, 250, 256
sleep-inducing breathing, 225–26
sleep inertia, 45, 81, 262, 265
sleep maintenance insomnia, 63, 245
Sleep Quality Index, 41
Sleep Regularity Index, 79–80
sleep-related breathing disorders, 69, 71.
    See also specific disorders
sleep-related movement disorders, 70
sleep rhythm, 22–23, 34
Sleep Science (journal), 18
sleep specialists, finding, 72
sleep spindles, 25
sleep study, 71, 72
sleep-tracking devices, 25, 27, 41, 45–48,
    245
sleepdoctor.com, 41, 244, 245
sleepwalking, 70
smoking, cigarette, 66, 228
snacking, pre-bedtime, 73
Šobat, Budimir, 175
social jet lag, 58, 61
soda, 65, 84, 118
sodium
    in hydration multiplier powders, 151
    hypothalamus and, 4, 101, 102
    overhydration and, 102, 131–32
    recommended daily allowance of, 151
    in water, 156, 157
    water retention and, 134, 138
Southeastern Lung Care, 8
spinach, 134, 155, 213
spinal cord, 100
spirometers, 182
spring water, 156–57, 162
standing, breathing and, 218, 233
Stanford University study, 194–95
static apnea, 175
steam, inhaling, 214–15
step counts, 269
Stone, Linda, 201
stress
    breathing and, 192, 203, 207–8, 221,
        226, 230
    heart rate variability and, 229

hydration and, 237
inflammation and, 189–90
sleep and, 28, 53–54, 92, 237
stress response, 9, 174, 203, 209, 222–23,
    227
stretching, 86, 254, 260, 267
stroke, 68, 190
    chronic inflammation and, 8, 143
    hydration and, 141, 143
    hypersomnia and, 62
    ischemic, at night, 29
    oxygen issues and, 200
    stress and, 208
Sunday night insomnia. *See* social jet lag
suprachiasmatic nucleus (SCN), 4
sweating
    humidity and, 88
    hydration and, 99, 102, 103, 106, 107,
        108, 131, 161
    sleeping and, 236
sympathetic nervous system, 33, 47, 86,
    189, 210
    breathing and, 190, 195, 208, 222
    heart rate variability and, 229
    hydrogen water and, 159

tanger, 72, 80
tap water, 135–37, 138, 156, 157, 245
Tap Water Database of Environmental
        Working Group, 135–36
tea, 65
    ginger, 215
    shifting, 84
    Sleep-Drink-Breathe Plan and
        Week 1, 250, 251, 253
        Week 2, 256, 257, 260
        Week 3, 263, 264, 267
teens, 36, 62, 198
teeth grinding, 70, 71
telomeres, 155, 210
temperature
    body, 4, 22, 85, 100, 106, 237
    climate, 88, 89, 147, 152, 244
testosterone, 81
thermogenesis, 142, 252, 258

thirst, 4, 113–14, 236
thirst cue, 104–5
Thirst Discomfort Scale, 113–14
thoracic breathing, 194
thyroid, overactive, 116
timeshifter.com, 71
Tiny Habits (Fogg), 150
toddlers, 36, 198
Tommy, 71n
total trihalomethanes, 136
trachea, 170, 171, 174, 212, 219, 238, 239
tunger, 52, 72, 78
turmeric, 230
Tylenol PM, 66–67

UCLA study, 50
ujjayi, 231
ulcers, 112
under-the-counter water filters, 157–58
underhydration, 103, 138
    bad habits responsible for, 128–30,
        132–35, *133*, 138, 149
    consequences of, 125–27, 138
University of Arkansas study, 127
University of Chicago study, 77–78
University of East London study, 143–44
University of Glasgow in Scotland study,
    148
urethra, 117, 119
Urinary Care Foundation, 117
urinary tract cancer, 112
urinary tract infections (UTIs). *See* UTIs
    (urinary tract infections)
urine
    cerebrospinal fluid and, 26
    color of, 101, *101*, 102, 110–12, 120
    frequency of, 115–18, 120, 121
    hydration and, 101, *101*, 102, 106,
        110–12, 132–33
    Sleep-Drink-Breathe Plan and, 247
        Week 1, 249, 250, 251, 252
        Week 2, 255, 256, 258
        Week 3, 262, 264, 266
    vasopressin and, 85
    volume of, 119–20, 121

U.S. Army Research Institute of
    Environmental Medicine, 145
USDA National Nutrient
    Database, 155
UTIs (urinary tract infections), 111
    dehydration and, 126, 129–30
    sexual activity and, 144
    urinary frequency and, 117, 121
    urinary volume and, 119, 120
    urine color and, 111, 112

vaginal dryness, 144
vagus nerve, 9, 207, 208, 225
vasopressin, 85, 101, 102, 118, 132, 135,
    160
vertical breathing, 196
vitamin A, 111, 135
vitamin B12, 111, 152
vitamin B6[13], 133
vitamin C, 135, 152, 213, 230
vitamin D, 71, 230
vitamin E, 213, 230
vitamin K, 135
vomiting, 103, 147, 152
vulva, 144

waking up, 4, 73
    chronotypes and, 81–82, 93, 243
    consistency in, 60, 81–82
    dehydration and, 132
    in middle-of-the-night, 63–64
    Sleep-Drink-Breathe Plan and, 242,
        243, 249–50, 255–56, 262–63
    on the weekends, 61
WatchPAT ONE kit, 41
water, 128
    alkaline, 159
    best choice of, for drinking, 156–57,
        162
    carbonated, 160
    contaminated, 135–37, 138
    content of foods, 155
    distilled, 157, 162, 214
    estimating water needs, 145–48,
        161–62

filters, 157–59
food and, 142, 154, 155, 162
hydrogen, 159–60
importance of, 99–100
infused with electrolytes, 124, 132, 147, 150–51
mineral, 140, 156, 162, 265
quenching, 104–5
retention, 134–35, 138
sharper cognition and, 143–44
Sleep-Drink-Breathe Plan and
    Week 1, 249, 250, 251, 252, 253
    Week 2, 255, 256, 257, 258–59, 260
    Week 3, 262, 264, 265, 266, 267, 268
spring, 156–57, 162
survival time without, 105–7, 108, 173
tap, 135–37, 138, 156, 157, 245
turnover rates of, 146
See also hydration
water intake, 85, 98, 99–102. *See also* hydration
water-salt ratio, 168
alcohol and, 118
caffeine and, 118
dehydration and, 124
overhydration and, 102, 131, 138
quenching and, 104
urine and, 111
water retention and, 134
water toxicity. *See* overhydration
watermelon, 135, 155

weight. *See* body weight
white blood cells, 50, 76, 143, 192
whole-body balance. *See* homeostasis
Whoop Strap, 46
Wim Hoff controlled hyperventilation method, 223, *223*
windpipe. *See* trachea
Winslet, Kate, 175
wolves (chronotype), 56–57, *57*
body mass index of, 56
cortisol of, 57, 238
dinner time of, 84
ideal bedtime of, 59, 82, 253, 259
ideal wake time of, 59, 81–82, 243, 249, 255, 262
inner alarms of, 58
napping and, 91
Sleep-Drink-Breathe Plan and, 243
    Week 1, 249, 250, 251, 252, 253
    Week 2, 255, 256, 257, 258, 259
    Week 3, 262, 263, 264, 266, 267
vigorous exercise and, 85

XPT (Extreme Performance Training), 169–70

yoga, 86, 124, 206, 207, 224, 231
yogic breathing, 206
young adults, 36, 62, 198

zolpidem, 66

about the author

Michael J. Breus, PhD, is a double board-certified clinical psychologist and clinical sleep specialist. He is one of only 168 psychologists in the world to have taken and passed the sleep medicine boards without going to medical school. Dr. Breus is the author of five books, including *Energize! Go from Dragging Ass to Kicking It in 30 Days*, named one of the top books of 2021 by the *Today Show*, and *The Power of When*, which is a groundbreaking biohacking book proving that there is a perfect time to do everything, based on your biological chronotype.

He is an expert resource for most major publications, doing more than four hundred interviews per year (Oprah, Dr. Oz, The Doctors, the *New York Times, Wall Street Journal*). Dr. Breus has been in private practice for nearly three decades and recently relocated to and was named the Top Sleep Doctor of Los Angeles by *Readers Digest*.

Find him at thesleepdoctor.com.